AF552626

Hormone Resistance and Hypersensitivity
From Genetics to Clinical Management

With an unrestricted educational grant from

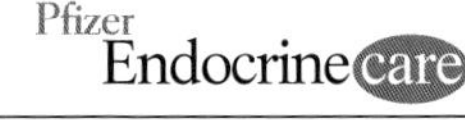

Endocrine Development

Vol. 24

Series Editor

P.-E. Mullis Bern

Workshop, May 13–15, 2012, Genoa, Italy

Hormone Resistance and Hypersensitivity

From Genetics to Clinical Management

Volume Editors

Mohamad Maghnie Genoa
Sandro Loche Cagliari
Marco Cappa Rome
Lucia Ghizzoni Turin
Renata Lorini Genoa

26 figures, 7 in color, and 10 tables, 2013

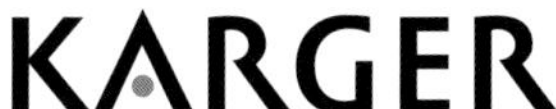

Basel · Freiburg · Paris · London · New York · New Delhi · Bangkok · Beijing · Tokyo · Kuala Lumpur · Singapore · Sydney

Endocrine Development
Founded 1999 by Martin O. Savage, London

Mohamad Maghnie
Department of Pediatrics
IRCCS G. Gaslini
University of Genoa
Genoa, Italy

Marco Cappa
Department of Pediatrics
Pediatric Hospital Bambino Gesù
Rome, Italy

Renata Lorini
Department of Pediatrics
IRCCS G. Gaslini
University of Genova
Genoa, Italy

Sandro Loche
Regional Hospital for
Microcytaemia
Cagliari, Italy

Lucia Ghizzoni
Division of Endocrinology
Diabetology and Metabolism
Department of Internal Medicine
University of Turin
Turin, Italy

Library of Congress Cataloging-in-Publication Data

Hormone resistance and hypersensitivity : from genetics to clinical management / volume editors, Mohamad Maghnie ... [et al.].
p. ; cm. -- (Endocrine development, ISSN 1421-7082 ; v. 24)
At head of title: Workshop, May 13-15, Genoa, Italy
"Meeting on hormone resistance and hypersensitivity - from genetics to clinical management held in Genoa, Italy, on May 13-15, 2012"--Pref.
Includes bibliographical references and indexes.
ISBN 978-3-318-02267-4 (hard cover : alk. paper) -- ISBN 978-3-318-02268-1 (electronic version)
I. Maghnie, Mohamad. II. Title: Workshop, May 13-15, Genoa, Italy. III. Series: Endocrine development ; v. 24. 1421-7082.
[DNLM: 1. Endocrine System Diseases--physiopathology--Congresses. 2. Hormones--metabolism--Congresses. 3. Hypersensitivity--genetics--Congresses. W1 EN3635 v.24 2013 / WK 140]

616.4'061--dc23

2012046360

Bibliographic Indices. This publication is listed in bibliographic services, including Current Contents®.

www.karger.com
Printed in Germany on acid-free and non-aging paper (ISO 97069) by Kraft Druck, Ettlingen
ISSN 1421–7082
e-ISSN 1662–2979
ISBN 978–3–318–02267–4
e-ISBN 978–3–318–02268–1

Contents

Preface

Over recent years, a tremendous progress has been made in the field of hormone resistance. The meeting on Hormone Resistance and Hypersensitivity – From Genetics to Clinical Management held in Genoa, Italy, on May 13–15, 2012, provided a unique opportunity for an updated and prospective view of this exciting topic.

The scientific program was designed to focus on the most recent advances related to the various aspects of hormone resistance affecting a number of endocrine or target organs. The impressive advances in genetic/epigenetic technology have greatly improved our understanding of the pathogenesis of pediatric endocrine diseases due to hormone resistance or hypersensitivity, as well as our diagnostic skills. Careful characterization of the phenotype of patients with hormone resistance together with decades of efforts in translational research have led to relevant improvements in the care of affected patients.

Hormone resistance is in fact a condition caused by a reduced or absent end-organ responsiveness to a biologically active hormone, which may be due to a hormone receptor defect (e.g. for glucocorticoids, androgens, estrogens, vitamin D derivatives, thyroid hormones, thyroid-stimulating hormone, parathyroid hormone, antidiuretic hormone, insulin) or a post-receptor defect. This book introduces clinical and genetic aspects of hormone resistance through a number of breakthrough developments that illustrate how molecular defects at various steps in hormone production, signaling, or responsiveness can cause disease in humans.

The volume contains reviews of thyroid hormone and thyroid hormone receptor resistance and genetics and epigenetics of parathyroid hormone resistance. Abnormalities of the pituitary-gonadal axis affecting puberty as well as androgen receptor are covered. We have broadened our understanding of the diseases affecting ACTH, glucocorticoid and aldosterone receptors. New aspects of the physiology of the GH and IGF-1 axis as well as the diseases related to GH-IGF-1 receptor and post-receptor signaling defects are comprehensively addressed.

A key chapter on metabolic insights into insulin resistance is also included.

Overall, this volume provides information directly useful to the clinician, and stimulates thought and future research opportunities with cutting-edge scientific results in the broad and important field of hormone resistance.

Mohamad Maghnie, Genoa
Sandro Loche, Cagliari
Marco Cappa, Rome
Lucia Ghizzoni, Turin
Renata Lorini, Genoa

Maghnie M, Loche S, Cappa M, Ghizzoni L, Lorini R (eds): Hormone Resistance and Hypersensitivity. From Genetics to Clinical Management. Endocr Dev. Basel, Karger, 2013, vol 24, pp 1–10 (DOI: 10.1159/000343695)

Thyroid Hormone Transporters and Resistance

Theo J. Visser

Department of Internal Medicine, Erasmus University Medical Center, Rotterdam, The Netherlands

Abstract

Cellular entry is an important step preceding intracellular metabolism and action of thyroid hormone (TH). Transport of TH across the plasma membrane does not take place by simple diffusion but requires transporter proteins. One of the most effective and specific TH transporters identified to date is monocarboxylate transporter 8 (MCT8), the gene of which is located on the X chromosome. Although MCT8 is expressed in many tissues, its function appears to be most critical in the brain. Hemizygous MCT8 mutations in males cause severe psychomotor retardation, known as the Allan-Herndon-Dudley syndrome (AHDS), and abnormal serum TH levels. AHDS thus represents a type of TH resistance caused by a defect in cellular TH transport.

The normal thyroid produces predominantly the prohormone thyroxine (3,3′,5,5′-tetraiodothyronine, T4) and only a small amount of the active hormone 3,3′,5-triiodothyronine (T3). Most T3 is generated by outer ring deiodination (ORD) of T4 in peripheral tissues [1]. In contrast, thyroid hormone (TH) is inactivated by inner ring deiodination (IRD), which converts T4 to 3,3′,5′-triiodothyronine (reverse T3, rT3) and T3 to 3,3′-diiodothyronine (3,3′-T2) [1].

TH is essential for the optimal development of different tissues, in particular the brain, as well as for the regulation of their basal metabolic rate throughout life. Most actions of TH are initiated by binding of T3 to nuclear T3 receptors (TRs). TRs are associated with T3 response elements in the promoter regions of T3 target genes usually as heterodimers with the retinoid X receptor. Binding of T3 results in a change in the interaction of TRs with associated proteins and consequently in an altered expression of the target genes [2–5].

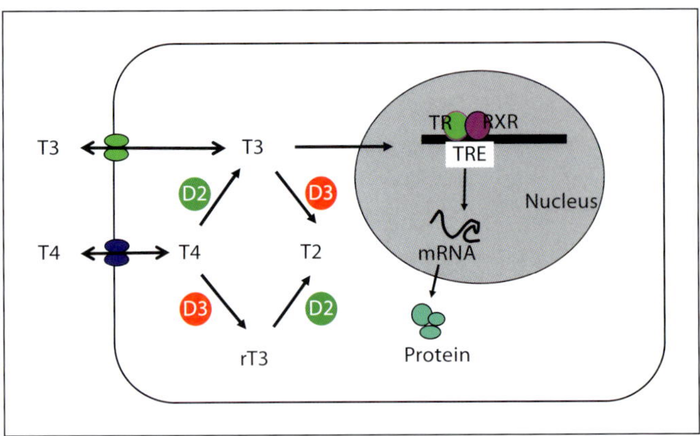

Fig. 1. Schematic of a TH target cell. The intracellular T3 concentration available for interaction with its nuclear receptor depends on (1) the circulating concentration of T3 and its precursor T4, (2) the activities of deiodinases which convert T4 to T3 (D2) or degrade T4 and T3 to inactive metabolites (D3), and (3) the expression of transporters which mediate the uptake and/or efflux of T3 and T4.

Two genes code for different TR isoforms: the *THRA* gene is located on human chromosome 17, and the *THRB* gene on human chromosome 3. Four major protein products are generated from these genes: TRα1, TRα2, TRβ1 and TRβ2. Through alternative splicing, TRα2 differs from TRα1 at the C-terminal ligand-binding domain and AF2 activation domain, and is unable to bind T3. The function of this receptor variant is uncertain. Through alternative exon usage, TRβ2 differs from TRβ1 at the N-terminus (AF1 activation domain). TRα1 and TRβ1 are widely expressed; TRα1 is predominant in brain, bone and heart, whereas TRβ1 is the major isoform in liver, kidney, and thyroid. TRβ2 has a more restricted expression pattern, regulating neurosensory development as well as the hypothalamus-pituitary-thyroid axis [2–5].

The biological activity of TH is thus largely determined by the intracellular T3 concentration, which is only indirectly dependent on the function of the thyroid gland. In many target tissues, T3 availability is regulated in a paracrine manner, where T3 supply to target cells is derived from T4 to T3 conversion in neighboring cells. Brain and cochlea are examples of tissues with paracrine regulation of TH action [3, 6–8]. In other tissues, such as the pituitary and brown adipose tissue, T3 may be produced from T4 directly in its target cells, representing an autocrine mechanism of TH action [1]. In yet other tissues such as the liver and the kidneys, intracellular T3 is in rapid exchange with circulating T3. This could be regarded as an endocrine action of T3, although it is still largely derived from peripheral conversion of T4 even in these same tissues [1].

The intracellular T3 concentration is dependent on three important factors: (1) the circulating concentrations of T3 and its precursor T4; (2) the activities of deiodinases that catalyze the activation of T4 to T3 or the degradation of T4 and T3 to inactive metabolites, and (3) the activity of transporters which mediate the uptake and/or efflux of T4 and T3 across the plasma membrane (fig. 1).

Three iodothyronine deiodinases (D1–3) are involved in the peripheral deiodination of TH, which are homologous selenoproteins containing a catalytic selenocysteine residue in their active centers [1]. D1 is highly expressed in the liver, kidney and thyroid. Although it has both ORD and IRD activity, it is thought to be an important site for serum T3 production. D2 has only ORD activity and is expressed in brain, pituitary, brown adipose tissue, thyroid and skeletal muscle. It is essential for local production of T3 in these tissues, but in particular the enzyme in the thyroid and muscle may also contribute to serum T3 production. D3 is highly expressed in different fetal tissues, placenta and pregnant uterus, and also in adult brain and skin. It has only IRD activity and thus plays a critical role in TH degradation. The deiodinases are integral membrane proteins embedded in the membrane of the endoplasmic reticulum or the plasma membrane such that the active sites are located in the cytoplasm [1].

Transport of TH across the plasma membrane does not take place by passive diffusion, but involves specific transporters [9, 10]. Various transporters have been identified which are capable of transporting TH among a wide variety of ligands. A notable exception is the organic anion transporting polypeptide 1C1 (OATP1C1), which is almost exclusively expressed in brain capillaries and shows a high specificity for T4 as the ligand. It is probably important for the transport of T4 across the blood-brain barrier [6, 8, 11–13]. Two other transporters, monocarboxylate transporter 8 (MCT8) and MCT10, have been characterized in our laboratory as effective TH transporters [14–16]. We and others have also demonstrated that mutations in MCT8 result in a syndrome combining severe psychomotor retardation and abnormal serum TH levels [17–20].

MCT8 and MCT10

The MCT family, now also known as the SLC16 family, contains 14 members. MCT1–4 facilitate uptake and/or efflux of monocarboxylates such as lactate and pyruvate [21]. MCT6 has been shown to transport the monocarboxylate drug bumetanide but physiological substrates have not been identified [22]. MCT7 has recently been characterized as an important efflux transporter for β-hydroxybutyrate [23]. MCT9 may transport uric acid and/or carnitine [24, 25], and MCT12 mutations result in cataract [26, 27]. The function of the other MCTs is unknown.

In 2001, MCT10 was identified as an aromatic amino acid transporter and named T-type amino acid transporter 1, which apparently lacked activity towards iodothyronines [28]. This led us to test its close homolog MCT8 for possible TH transport, which was indeed found to be the case [14, 16]. We have later shown that – in contrast to the initially negative results – MCT10 is a very effective TH transporter [15].

MCT8 and *MCT10* have similar gene structures. *MCT8* is located on human chr X13.2 and *MCT10* on chr 6q21-q22. Both genes have 6 exons and, thus, 5 introns with a particularly large first intron (~100 kb). Human *MCT8* has two possible translation start sites (TLSs), yielding a larger protein of 613 amino acids or a shorter protein of

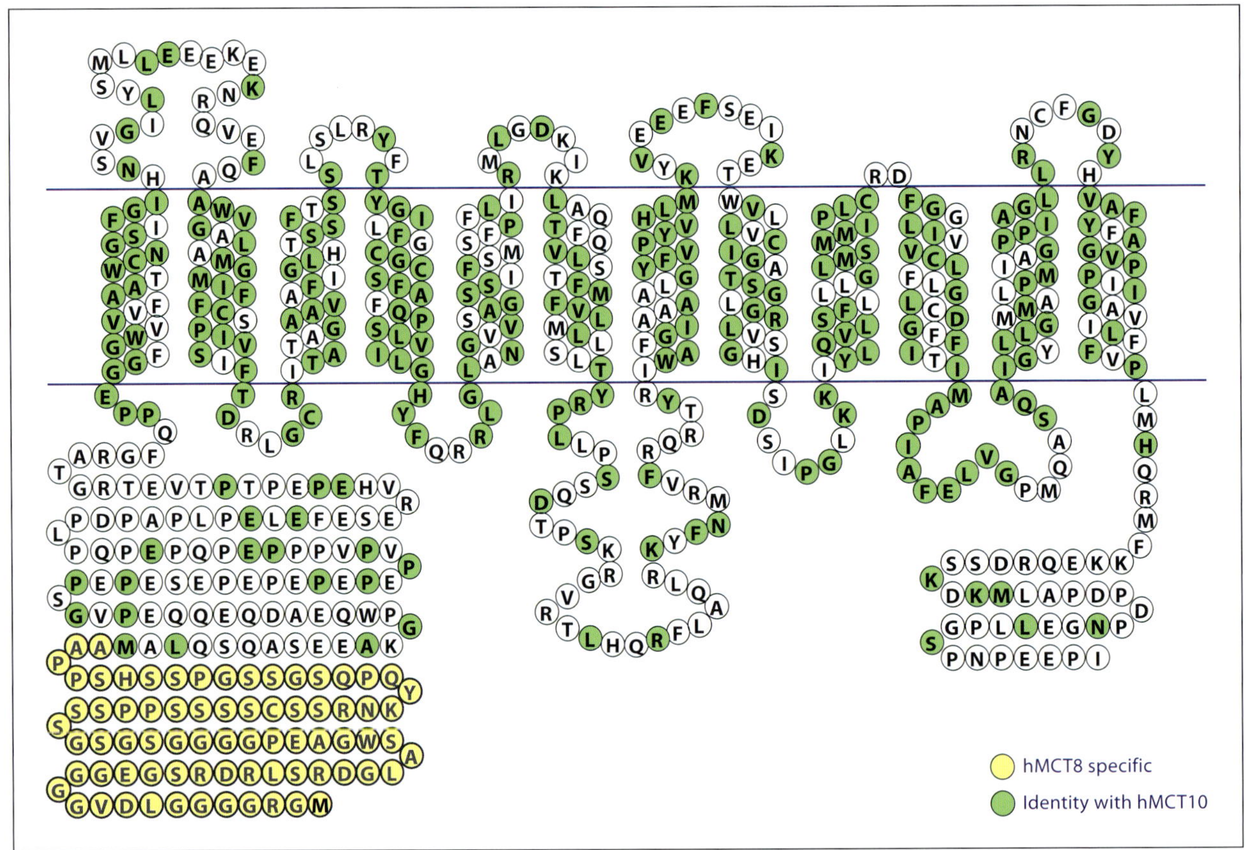

Fig. 2. Protein structure of human MCT8 and amino acid identity with human MCT10.

539 amino acids (fig. 2). In many animals, *MCT8* lacks the first TLS and thus codes only for the short MCT8 protein. The possible function of the N-terminal extension of the long human MCT8 protein, if any, remains to be determined. In all species, *MCT10* has only one TLS, corresponding to the second TLS of human MCT8, coding for a protein of 515 amino acids.

MCT8 and MCT10 have 12 putative transmembrane domains (TMDs); both N-and C-terminal domains are located intracellularly [14–16]. There is a high degree of homology between the MCT8 and MCT10 proteins, in particular in the TMDs, which corresponds with the similar functions of these proteins. Both MCT8 and MCT10 facilitate transport of different iodothyronines, although T3 is transported somewhat better by MCT10 than by MCT8, whereas T4 is clearly a better ligand for MCT8 than for MCT10 [15, 16]. Both MCT8 and MCT10 facilitate cellular uptake as well as efflux of iodothyronines. Therefore, transfection of cells with MCT8 or MCT10 may only result in a modest increase in steady-state intracellular TH levels in the presence of endogenous TH transporters. Net TH uptake is markedly increased

Neurological findings	Central hypotonia, poor head control Distal hypotonia progressing to spastic quadriplegia Inability to sit, stand, walk
Mental development	Severe retardation
Speech development	None
Physical	Reduced body length Very low bodyweight Progressive microcephaly
Brain MRI	Delayed myelination
Serum thyroid parameters	Low T4, high T3 Modest increase in TSH

Fig. 3. Characteristics of AHDS.

if efflux is inhibited for instance by cotransfection with the cytoplasmic TH-binding protein μ-crystallin [15]. MCT8 and MCT10 indeed increase intracellular TH availability as demonstrated by the marked increase in TH metabolism by D1, D2 or D3 in cells cotransfected with these transporters [15, 16].

MCT8 and MCT10 are expressed in many human tissues. MCT8 is highly expressed in the liver, kidney, adrenal, ovary and thyroid [29]. As demonstrated by studies in mice, MCT8 is also expressed importantly in brain, in particular in neurons in different brain regions, including cerebral cortex and cerebellum, but also in the choroid plexus, in capillaries and in tanycytes lining the 3rd ventricle [6–8]. MCT10 shows particularly high expression in skeletal muscle, intestine and kidney [29].

Patients with MCT8 Mutations

The pathophysiological importance of MCT8 has been established by studies in male patients with severe psychomotor retardation and abnormal serum TH levels caused by hemizygous MCT8 mutations [17–20]. The neurological syndrome has already been described in 1944 [30], and since then named after the authors as the Allan-Herndon-Dudley syndrome (AHDS). A detailed description of AHDS has been published more recently [31]. It comprises central hypotonia associated with poor head control and initially also peripheral hypotonia that progresses to spasticity (fig. 3). Most AHDS patients are unable to sit, stand or walk independently; neither have they acquired speech. However, some less severely affected patients have been reported who are able to walk and/or talk with great difficulty. All patients have severe mental retardation, although again there is some phenotypic variation [31]. AHDS is often not apparent at birth and develops progressively, frequently associated with microcephaly. MRI of the brain usually shows delayed myelination before the age of 2 years which apparently normalizes with increasing age [20].

In addition to the psychomotor retardation, AHDS patients also show abnormal serum thyroid parameters [17–20]. Serum T4 and FT4 levels vary from low-normal to actually decreased, whereas serum T3 levels are invariably increased. Like T4, serum rT3 is usually decreased, and the serum T3/rT3 ratio is markedly elevated. Serum TSH varies between normal and elevated; mean TSH levels are about twice the normal mean. In view of the low serum FT4 and somewhat higher TSH levels, many AHDS patients have received LT4 substitution therapy without obvious benefit.

TH is crucial for brain development [32]. However, in AHDS patients, brain development is impaired despite the presence of high serum T3 levels, suggesting some form of TH resistance. Initial studies indicated that this was not caused by mutations in one of the TRs or deiodinases. It was then hypothesized that TH resistance in AHDS patients is caused by impaired TH uptake in target cells due to mutations in a TH transporter. Since AHDS only occurs in males and *MCT8* is located on the X chromosome, the hypothesis was tested by analysis of the *MCT8* sequence for possible mutations. Indeed, in over 50 families with AHDS studied so far, various mutations in *MCT8* have been identified [33].

MCT8 mutations identified in AHDS patients include large deletions, frameshift mutations and non-sense mutations, which are obviously deleterious for MCT8 function. However, this is not so obvious for mutations that result in the deletion, insertion or substitutions of single amino acids. The functional consequences of these more subtle mutations have been tested by analysis of TH uptake and metabolism in cells transfected with wild-type (WT) or mutated MCT8. All mutations result in a marked decrease in TH transport, although the magnitude of the defect depends on the cell type used for in vitro analyses [34–36]. Defective cellular TH uptake has also been demonstrated using fibroblast from AHDS patients in comparison with fibroblasts from healthy subjects [37]. In general, the findings suggest some correlation between the severity of the clinical phenotype, the changes in serum TH levels and the defect in TH transport.

The pathogenic mechanism of AHDS involves an important role of MCT8 in T3 uptake in central neurons and, hence, in the crucial action of T3 in this important target cell during brain development. Inactivation of MCT8 results in the lack of T3 supply to its nuclear receptor in these neurons and, thus, in impaired differentiation of these cells, with dramatic consequences for brain development [38]. However, MCT8 is also highly expressed in endothelial cells and the choroid plexus [6–8]. Therefore, it may also play an important role in brain TH uptake at the blood-brain barrier as well as the blood-cerebrospinal fluid barrier.

Animal Model

To study the pathogenic mechanism of MCT8 mutations in more detail, *Mct8* knockout (KO) mice have been studied in different laboratories [39–41]. Surprisingly, Mct8

KO mice do not show any remarkable neurological phenotype. They do show, however, the same decrease in serum T4 and increase in T3 levels as AHDS patients. Studies into the mechanism(s) underlying the altered serum TH levels have indicated (a) increased D1 expression in liver and kidney, (b) increased D2 activity in brain and pituitary, and (c) decreased D3 activity in brain of Mct8 KO versus WT animals [40, 42].

The important role of MCT8 in brain TH transport is evident from the almost complete block in T3 uptake in Mct8 KO mice, whereas T4 uptake is hardly affected [40]. T4 and T3 uptake in the liver is not inhibited in Mct8 KO mice while, unexpectedly, T4 and T3 appear to accumulate at higher levels in kidneys form Mct8 KO mice than in WT mice [40, 42]. This surprising finding may be explained if MCT8 is more important for TH efflux than for TH uptake in the kidney. The increased tissue T4 content in combination with the higher D1 activity in the kidney may contribute to a strong increase in peripheral T4 to T3 conversion, and, thus, to the low T4 and high serum T3 levels in MCT8-deficient subjects [42].

One of the most remarkable findings in Mct8 KO mice concerns the important role of MCT8 in TH secretion [43, 44]. Thyroidal T4 and T3 content is higher in Mct8 KO than in WT mice. Furthermore, after stimulation of mice with TSH, the increase in serum T4 is lower, whereas the increase in serum T3 is higher in Mct8 KO than in WT mice [44]. This suggests that T4 secretion from thyroid cells is mediated importantly by MCT8. If MCT8 is inactivated, T4 accumulates in the thyrocyte, leading to increased intrathyroidal T4 to T3 conversion, and thus an increase in the ratio of secreted T3 versus T4.

It is difficult to decide if the somewhat higher serum TSH levels in AHDS patients than in healthy controls are appropriate or not in view of the decreased serum T4 and increased T3 levels. MCT8 is highly expressed in different cell types in the hypothalamus, and may thus be involved in the negative feedback of TH at the hypothalamus [45, 46]. This is in agreement with the reduced potency of injected T3 to suppress TRH expression in MCT8 KO compared with WT mice [44].

TH Resistance Caused by Receptor Mutations

Numerous patients have been reported with resistance to TH (RTH) caused by heterozygous mutations in *THRB*. Extensive reviews have been published on this subject [47, 48]. The mutations are usually located in the ligand-binding domain of TRβ1 and TRβ2, resulting in a partial or complete loss of T3 binding affinity. The mutated receptor has a dominant-negative effect on the activity of the WT receptor.

Since the negative feedback of T3 at both the hypothalamus and the pituitary is mediated by TRβ2, RTH patients exhibit increased serum T4 and T3 levels in the presence of non-suppressed TSH levels. Depending on the possible compensation of the receptor defect by the increased serum T3 levels, tissues with predominant TRβ expression are in a euthyroid or hypothyroid state. However, tissues with predominant TRα expression may be in a hyperthyroid state as this normally functioning receptor is exposed to elevated T3 concentrations. Tachycardia, atrial fibrillation and osteoporosis are therefore observed in a significant number of RTH patients, reflecting the excessive action of TH in the heart and bone. Other symptoms may include goiter and mild mental retardation.

Ever since its characterization in 1987, investigators have searched for patients with mutations in *THRA*. As TRα1 is not involved in the negative feedback action of TH, no major changes in serum TH levels were expected. Even TRα1 mutant mouse models have been developed to predict the clinical phenotype in patients with *THRA* mutations [49]. Only very recently, 3 patients have been reported with inactivating mutations in TRα1 [50, 51]. All patients showed marked growth retardation, markedly delayed bone development, mildly delayed motor and mental development, and constipation. These symptoms appear to reflect the important roles of TRα1 in bone, brain and intestine. In addition, the patients showed low serum T4, high T3 and normal TSH levels. These changes are similar to those seen in patients with *MCT8* mutations. The mechanisms underlying these changes in serum TH levels may involve impaired expression of D3, the enzyme which degrades TH with a substrate preference for T3. D3 expression is stimulated by T3, and this regulation is specifically mediated by TRα1 [52].

References

1 Gereben B, Zavacki AM, Ribich S, Kim BW, Huang SA, Simonides WS, Zeold A, Bianco AC: Cellular and molecular basis of deiodinase-regulated thyroid hormone signaling. Endocr Rev 2008;29:898–938.

2 Cheng SY, Leonard JL, Davis PJ: Molecular aspects of thyroid hormone actions. Endocr Rev 2010;31: 139–170.

3 Nunez J, Celi FS, Ng L, Forrest D: Multigenic control of thyroid hormone functions in the nervous system. Mol Cell Endocrinol 2008;287:1–12.

4 Yen PM: Physiological and molecular basis of thyroid hormone action. Physiol Rev 2001;81: 1097–1142.

5 Wojcicka A, Bassett JH, Williams GR: Mechanisms of action of thyroid hormones in the skeleton. Biochim Biophys Acta 2012, Epub ahead of print.

6 Bernal J: Thyroid hormone transport in developing brain. Curr Opin Endocrinol Diabetes Obes 2011; 18:295–299.

7 Heuer H: The importance of thyroid hormone transporters for brain development and function. Best Pract Res 2007;21:265–276.

8 Schweizer U, Kohrle J: Function of thyroid hormone transporters in the central nervous system. Biochim Biophys Acta 2012, Epub ahead of print.

9 Hennemann G, Docter R, Friesema EC, de Jong M, Krenning EP, Visser TJ: Plasma membrane transport of thyroid hormones and its role in thyroid hormone metabolism and bioavailability. Endocr Rev 2001;22:451–476.

10 Visser WE, Friesema EC, Visser TJ: Minireview: thyroid hormone transporters: the knowns and the unknowns. Mol Endocrinol (Baltimore) 2011;25: 1–14.

11 Heuer H, Visser TJ: Minireview: pathophysiological importance of thyroid hormone transporters. Endocrinology 2009;150:1078–1083.

12 Pizzagalli F, Hagenbuch B, Stieger B, Klenk U, Folkers G, Meier PJ: Identification of a novel human organic anion transporting polypeptide as a high affinity thyroxine transporter. Mol Endocrinol (Baltimore) 2002;16:2283–2296.

13 Roberts LM, Woodford K, Zhou M, Black DS, Haggerty JE, Tate EH, Grindstaff KK, Mengesha W, Raman C, Zerangue N: Expression of the thyroid hormone transporters MCT8 (SLC16A2) and OATP14 (SLCO1C1) at the blood-brain barrier. Endocrinology 2008;149:6251–6261.

14 Friesema EC, Ganguly S, Abdalla A, Manning Fox JE, Halestrap AP, Visser TJ: Identification of monocarboxylate transporter 8 as a specific thyroid hormone transporter. J Biol Chem 2003;278: 40128–40135.

15 Friesema EC, Jansen J, Jachtenberg JW, Visser WE, Kester MH, Visser TJ: Effective cellular uptake and efflux of thyroid hormone by human monocarboxylate transporter 10. Mol Endocrinol (Baltimore) 2008;22:1357–1369.

16 Friesema EC, Kuiper GG, Jansen J, Visser TJ, Kester MH: Thyroid hormone transport by the human monocarboxylate transporter 8 and its rate-limiting role in intracellular metabolism. Mol Endocrinol (Baltimore) 2006;20:2761–2772.

17 Dumitrescu AM, Liao XH, Best TB, Brockmann K, Refetoff S: A novel syndrome combining thyroid and neurological abnormalities is associated with mutations in a monocarboxylate transporter gene. Am J Hum Genet 2004;74:168–175.

18 Friesema EC, Grueters A, Biebermann H, Krude H, von Moers A, Reeser M, Barrett TG, Mancilla EE, Svensson J, Kester MH, Kuiper GG, Balkassmi S, Uitterlinden AG, Koehrle J, Rodien P, Halestrap AP, Visser TJ: Association between mutations in a thyroid hormone transporter and severe X-linked psychomotor retardation. Lancet 2004;364:1435–1437.

19 Schwartz CE, May MM, Carpenter NJ, Rogers RC, Martin J, Bialer MG, Ward J, Sanabria J, Marsa S, Lewis JA, Echeverri R, Lubs HA, Voeller K, Simensen RJ, Stevenson RE: Allan-Herndon-Dudley syndrome and the monocarboxylate transporter 8 (MCT8) gene. Am J Hum Genet 2005; 77:41–53.

20 Vaurs-Barriere C, Deville M, Sarret C, Giraud G, Des Portes V, Prats-Vinas JM, De Michele G, Dan B, Brady AF, Boespflug-Tanguy O, Touraine R: Pelizaeus-Merzbacher-Like disease presentation of MCT8 mutated male subjects. Ann Neurol 2009; 65:114–118.

21 Halestrap AP, Meredith D: The SLC16 gene family-from monocarboxylate transporters (MCTs) to aromatic amino acid transporters and beyond. Pflugers Arch 2004;447:619–628.

22 Murakami Y, Kohyama N, Kobayashi Y, Ohbayashi M, Ohtani H, Sawada Y, Yamamoto T: Functional characterization of human monocarboxylate transporter 6 (SLC16A5). Drug metabolism and disposition: the biological fate of chemicals 2005;33: 1845–1851.

23 Hugo SE, Cruz-Garcia L, Karanth S, Anderson RM, Stainier DY, Schlegel A: A monocarboxylate transporter required for hepatocyte secretion of ketone bodies during fasting. Genes Dev 2012;26:282–293.

24 Illig T, Gieger C, Zhai G, Romisch-Margl W, Wang-Sattler R, Prehn C, Altmaier E, Kastenmuller G, Kato BS, Mewes HW, Meitinger T, de Angelis MH, Kronenberg F, Soranzo N, Wichmann HE, Spector TD, Adamski J, Suhre K: A genome-wide perspective of genetic variation in human metabolism. Nat Genet 2010;42:137–141.

25 Kolz M, Johnson T, Sanna S, et al: Meta-analysis of 28,141 individuals identifies common variants within five new loci that influence uric acid concentrations. PLoS Genet 2009;5:e1000504.

26 Castorino JJ, Gallagher-Colombo SM, Levin AV, Fitzgerald PG, Polishook J, Kloeckener-Gruissem B, Ostertag E, Philp NJ: Juvenile cataract-associated mutation of solute carrier SLC16A12 impairs trafficking of the protein to the plasma membrane. Invest Ophthalmol Vis Sci 2012;52:6774–6784.

27 Kloeckener-Gruissem B, Vandekerckhove K, Nurnberg G, Neidhardt J, Zeitz C, Nurnberg P, Schipper I, Berger W: Mutation of solute carrier SLC16A12 associates with a syndrome combining juvenile cataract with microcornea and renal glucosuria. Am J Hum Genet 2008;82:772–779.

28 Kim DK, Kanai Y, Chairoungdua A, Matsuo H, Cha SH, Endou H: Expression cloning of a Na^+-independent aromatic amino acid transporter with structural similarity to H^+/monocarboxylate transporters. J Biol Chem 2001;276:17221–17228.

29 Nishimura M, Naito S: Tissue-specific mRNA expression profiles of human solute carrier transporter superfamilies. Drug Metab Pharmacokinet 2008;23:22–44.

30 Allan W, Herndon CN, Dudley FC: Some examples of the inheritance of mental deficiency: apparently sex-linked idiocy and microcephaly. Am J Mental Defic 1944;48:325–334.

31 Holden KR, Zuniga OF, May MM, Su H, Molinero MR, Rogers RC, Schwartz CE: X-linked MCT8 gene mutations: characterization of the pediatric neurologic phenotype. J Child Neurol 2005;20:852–857.

32 Bernal J: Thyroid hormone receptors in brain development and function. Nat Clin Pract 2007;3: 249–259.

33 Friesema EC, Visser WE, Visser TJ: Genetics and phenomics of thyroid hormone transport by MCT8. Mol Cell Endocrinol 2010;322:107–113.

34 Jansen J, Friesema EC, Kester MH, Milici C, Reeser M, Gruters A, Barrett TG, Mancilla EE, Svensson J, Wemeau JL, Busi da Silva Canalli MH, Lundgren J, McEntagart ME, Hopper N, Arts WF, Visser TJ: Functional analysis of monocarboxylate transporter 8 mutations identified in patients with x-linked psychomotor retardation and elevated serum triiodothyronine. J Clin Endocrinol Metab 2007;92:2378–2381.
35 Jansen J, Friesema EC, Kester MH, Schwartz CE, Visser TJ: Genotype-phenotype relationship in patients with mutations in thyroid hormone transporter MCT8. Endocrinology 2008;149:2184–2190.
36 Kinne A, Roth S, Biebermann H, Koehrle J, Gruters A, Schweizer U: Surface translocation and T3 uptake of mutant MCT8 proteins are cell type-dependent. J Mol Endocrinol 2009;43:263–271.
37 Visser WE, Philp NJ, van Dijk TB, Klootwijk W, Friesema EC, Jansen J, Beesley PW, Ianculescu AG, Visser TJ: Evidence for a homodimeric structure of human monocarboxylate transporter 8. Endocrinology 2009;150:5163–5170.
38 Friesema EC, Jansen J, Heuer H, Trajkovic M, Bauer K, Visser TJ: Mechanisms of disease: psychomotor retardation and high T3 levels caused by mutations in monocarboxylate transporter 8. Nat Clin Pract 2006;2:512–523.
39 Dumitrescu AM, Liao XH, Weiss RE, Millen K, Refetoff S: Tissue-specific thyroid hormone deprivation and excess in monocarboxylate transporter (mct) 8-deficient mice. Endocrinology 2006;147:4036–4043.
40 Trajkovic M, Visser TJ, Mittag J, Horn S, Lukas J, Darras VM, Raivich G, Bauer K, Heuer H: Abnormal thyroid hormone metabolism in mice lacking the monocarboxylate transporter 8. J Clin Invest 2007;117:627–635.
41 Wirth EK, Roth S, Blechschmidt C, Holter SM, Becker L, Racz I, Zimmer A, Klopstock T, Gailus-Durner V, Fuchs H, Wurst W, Naumann T, Brauer A, de Angelis MH, Kohrle J, Gruters A, Schweizer U: Neuronal 3′,3,5-triiodothyronine (T3) uptake and behavioral phenotype of mice deficient in Mct8, the neuronal T3 transporter mutated in Allan-Herndon-Dudley syndrome. J Neurosci 2009; 29:9439–9449.
42 Trajkovic M, Visser TJ, Darras WM, Friesema ECH, Schlott B, Mittag J, Bauer K, Heuer H: Consequences of MCT8 deficiency for renal transport and metabolism of thyroid hormones in mice. Endocrinology 2009;151:802–809.
43 Di Cosmo C, Liao XH, Dumitrescu AM, Philp NJ, Weiss RE, Refetoff S: Mice deficient in MCT8 reveal a mechanism regulating thyroid hormone secretion. J Clin Invest 2010;120:3377–3388.
44 Trajkovic-Arsic M, Müller J, Darras VM, Groba C, Lee S, Weih D, Bauer K, Visser TJ, Heuer H: Impact of monocarboxylate transporter (Mct)-8 deficiency on the hypothalamus-pituitary-thyroid axis in mice. Endocrinology 2010;151:5053–5062.
45 Alkemade A, Friesema EC, Kalsbeek A, Swaab DF, Visser TJ, Fliers E: Expression of thyroid hormone transporters in the human hypothalamus. J Clin Endocrinol Metab 2011;96:E967–E971.
46 Heuer H, Maier MK, Iden S, Mittag J, Friesema EC, Visser TJ, Bauer K: The monocarboxylate transporter 8 linked to human psychomotor retardation is highly expressed in thyroid hormone-sensitive neuron populations. Endocrinology 2005;146:1701–1706.
47 Refetoff S, Dumitrescu AM: Syndromes of reduced sensitivity to thyroid hormone: genetic defects in hormone receptors, cell transporters and deiodination. Best Pract Res 2007;21:277–305.
48 Yen PM: Molecular basis of resistance to thyroid hormone. Trends Endocrinol Metab 2003;14:327–333.
49 Vennstrom B, Mittag J, Wallis K: Severe psychomotor and metabolic damages caused by a mutant thyroid hormone receptor alpha 1 in mice: can patients with a similar mutation be found and treated? Acta Paediatr 2008;97:1605–1610.
50 Bochukova E, Schoenmakers N, Agostini M, et al: A mutation in the thyroid hormone receptor alpha gene. N Engl J Med 2012;366:243–249.
51 van Mullem A, van Heerebeek R, Chrysis D, Visser E, Medici M, Andrikoula M, Tsatsoulis A, Peeters R, Visser TJ: Clinical phenotype and mutant TRalpha1. N Engl J Med 2012;366:1451–1453.
52 Barca-Mayo O, Liao XH, Alonso M, Di Cosmo C, Hernandez A, Refetoff S, Weiss RE: Thyroid hormone receptor alpha and regulation of type 3 deiodinase. Mol Endocrinol (Baltimore) 2011;25:575–583.

Theo J. Visser
Department of Internal Medicine
Erasmus University Medical Center
NL–3015 GE Rotterdam (The Netherlands)
E-Mail t.j.visser@erasmusmc.nl

Maghnie M, Loche S, Cappa M, Ghizzoni L, Lorini R (eds): Hormone Resistance and Hypersensitivity. From Genetics to Clinical Management. Endocr Dev. Basel, Karger, 2013, vol 24, pp 11–24 (DOI: 10.1159/000342494)

Genetics and Epigenetics of Parathyroid Hormone Resistance

Murat Bastepe

Endocrine Unit, Department of Medicine, Massachusetts General Hospital and Harvard Medical School, Boston, Mass., USA

Abstract

End-organ resistance to the actions of parathyroid hormone (PTH) is defined as pseudohypoparathyroidism (PHP). Described originally by Fuller Albright and his colleagues in early 1940s, this rare genetic disease is subclassified into two types according to the nephrogenous response to the administration of biologically active PTH. In type I, the PTH-induced urinary excretion of both phosphate and cyclic AMP (cAMP) is blunted. In type II, only the PTH-induced urinary excretion of phosphate is blunted, while the cAMP response is unimpaired. Different subtypes of PHP type I have been described based on the existence of additional clinical features, such as resistance to other hormones and Albright's hereditary osteodystrophy, and underlying molecular defects. Genetic mutations responsible for the different subtypes of PHP type I involve the *GNAS* complex locus, an imprinted gene encoding the α-subunit of the stimulatory G protein (Gsα) and several other transcripts that are expressed in a parent-of-origin specific manner. Mutations in Gsα-coding *GNAS* exons cause PHP-Ia and, in some cases, PHP-Ic, while mutations that disrupt the imprinting of *GNAS* lead to PHP-Ib. PHP type II is less well characterized with respect to its molecular cause. Recently, however, mutations in PRKAR1A, a regulatory subunit of the cAMP-dependent protein kinase, have been identified in several cases of PTH and other hormone resistance and skeletal dysplasia that are considered to be affected by PHP type II due to unimpaired urinary excretion of cAMP following PTH administration.

Parathyroid hormone (PTH) is one of the key molecules that act on bone and kidney to regulate calcium and phosphate homeostasis. In bone, PTH increases bone turnover and leads to the mobilization of bone mineral into the circulation. In the renal proximal tubule, PTH stimulates the synthesis of the biologically active form of vitamin D, i.e. 1,25 dihydroxy vitamin D, and inhibits the reabsorption of phosphate from the glomerular filtrate. PTH also acts on the distal portion of the nephron, where it enhances the reabsorption of calcium from the filtrate. End-organ resistance to the actions of PTH, which primarily occurs in the renal proximal tubule, is termed pseudohypoparathyroidism (PHP). This disorder was described first in 1942 by Albright

Table 1. Clinical as well as genetic and epigenetic features associated with the different types and subtypes of PHP

	PTH-induced urinary phosphate	PTH-induced urinary cAMP	PTH resistance	TSH resistance	Other hormone resistance	AHO	Genetic defect
PHP type I	blunted	blunted					
PHP-Ia			yes	yes	yes	yes	Gsα coding (het. inactivating)
PPHP			no	no	no	yes	Gsα coding (het. inactivating)
PHP-Ic			yes	yes	yes	yes	Gsα coding (het. receptor unc.)
PHP-Ib (familial)			yes	yes (some)	no	no	*GNAS* imprinting defects; het. *STX16* deletions; het. NESP55 DMR or antisense exon deletions
PHP-Ib (sporadic)			yes	yes (some)	no	no	*GNAS* imprinting defects; patUPD20; unknown
PHP type II	blunted	normal	yes	yes	yes	yes	PRKAR1A (het. preventing PKA activation)

het. = Heterozygous; unc. = uncoupling; patUPD20 = paternal uniparental disomy of chromosome 20.

et al. [1], who reported several patients exhibiting a number of physical and skeletal defects, now collectively termed Albright's hereditary osteodystrophy (AHO), as well as hypocalcemia and hyperphosphatemia that were resistant to exogenously administered biologically active PTH. Two main types of PHP have since been described (table 1): patients with PHP type I show a blunted response to exogenously administered PTH with respect to the urinary excretion of both phosphate and cyclic AMP (cAMP), whereas patients with PHP type II show a blunted response only regarding the PTH-induced urinary excretion of phosphate [1–3].

Although a part of the original description of PHP, AHO is present only in a certain group of patients with PTH resistance, who are now said to be affected by PHP type Ia (PHP-Ia). In addition to AHO and PTH resistance, patients with this PHP subtype show end-organ resistance to additional hormones, including thyroid-stimulating hormone (TSH), gonadotropins, and growth hormone-releasing hormone [4–10]. Together with PTH, all of these hormones exert their actions by binding to cell surface receptors that couple to the stimulatory heterotrimeric G protein. Accordingly, PHP-Ia is caused by heterozygous inactivating mutations in the gene encoding the α-subunit of this G protein (Gsα) [11, 12]. Gsα is encoded by *GNAS*, which is located on the telomeric end of chromosome 20q (20q13.3) [13–16]. Mutations identified in PHP-Ia patients can be found in all the 13 exons that encode Gsα and range from missense and non-sense mutations to different types of deletions, and to large deletions that remove the genomic region comprising the whole or part of *GNAS*.

The stimulatory G protein is a signaling protein that mediates, through generation of the second messenger cAMP, the actions of a whole host of endogenous molecules, including many hormones, neurotransmitters, and autocrine/paracrine factors [reviewed in references 17–19]. In spite of the diversity of actions mediated by this ubiquitously expressed protein, the clinical features of patients with PHP-Ia are relatively limited, particularly with respect to hormone resistance. While the actions of some hormones that act via Gsα-coupled receptors are impaired, the actions of many other molecules that also utilize Gsα in their signaling, such as vasopressin and adrenocorticoptropic hormone, are seemingly unimpaired [9, 20–22]. In addition, the same *GNAS* mutations that cause PHP-Ia are found in some patients who lack hormone resistance but show features of AHO, a disorder termed pseudo-pseudohypoparathyroidism (PPHP) [23]. PHP-Ia and PPHP are frequently present in the same kindreds, but never in the same sibship. When a Gsα mutation is inherited from the mother, the offspring develops AHO together with hormone resistance, i.e. PHP-Ia. In contrast, when the same mutation is inherited from the father, the offspring develops AHO alone, i.e. PPHP [24]. The limited nature of hormonal impairments and the parent-of-origin specific inheritance of the hormone resistance can be explained by the fact that Gsα expression occurs predominantly from the maternal *GNAS* allele in a small subset of tissues, including renal proximal tubules, thyroid, gonads, pituitary, and certain parts of the brain [25–31]. In other words, the paternal Gsα allele is silenced in these tissues. Gsα expression is biallelic in most other tissues [32–37]. Thus, in tissues in which Gsα expression is predominantly maternal, a *GNAS* mutation located on the maternal allele leads to a dramatic reduction in Gsα expression/activity, whereas the same *GNAS* mutation located on the paternal allele does not result in a significant change.

Based on the original description, AHO includes obesity, short stature, brachydactyly, ectopic ossification, and cognitive impairment [1]. However, recent studies have shown that obesity and cognitive impairment develop primarily upon maternal inheritance of *GNAS* mutations [38, 39], consistent with the predominant maternal expression of Gsα in certain parts of the brain [31]. In broad terms, it is accepted that AHO features develop regardless of the parental origin of a *GNAS* mutation, and therefore, it is thought that these features result from Gsα haploinsufficiency in various tissues in which Gsα expression is biallelic. Supporting this hypothesis, heterozygous loss of either the maternal or the paternal Gsα allele leads to acceleration of the hypertrophic differentiation of growth plate chondrocytes [37]. The Gsα haploinsufficiency in this setting likely contributes to the brachydactyly and the short stature observed in patients with AHO.

In erythrocytes derived from patients with PHP-Ia and PPHP, Gsα expression/bioactivity is reduced by approximately 50%, and the measurement of Gsα bioactivity in these cells is utilized as a diagnostic method [4, 40–52]. Typically, membranes from patient-derived erythrocytes are reconstituted with turkey erythrocytes that lack endogenous Gsα, and cAMP levels are measured in response to different stimuli. Some patients that clinically appear as PHP-Ia patients, i.e. multihormone resistance and AHO, have shown apparently normal Gsα bioactivity in this reconstitution assay, leading to the definition of PHP-Ic [43] (table 1). The normal Gsα bioactivity in these patients may indicate that the molecular defect is downstream of Gsα. However, at least in a subset of PHP-Ic patients, heterozygous *GNAS* mutations have been identified, and it has been shown that these mutations impair receptor-dependent but not receptor-independent cAMP formation, i.e. the mutant Gsα protein is uncoupled from the receptor but is otherwise able to stimulate cAMP synthesis [53, 54]. The Gsα bioactivity appears normal in these PHP-Ic cases when cAMP generation in the complementation assay is induced by agents that activate Gsα directly, such as GTP analogs. Generation of cAMP is blunted, however, when receptor agonists are utilized [54, 55].

PHP-Ib is another subtype of PHP type I characterized by hormone resistance in the absence of AHO [56, 57] (table 1). The hormone resistance is primarily limited to PTH in patients with PHP-Ib, but mild resistance to TSH is also observed frequently [27, 58–60]. In contrast to PHP-Ia, resistance to gonadotropins has not been reported, and resistance to GHRH was observed only in one of 10 cases analyzed in that regard [60]. A Gsα mutation in exon 13 (deletion of Ile382) has been reported in three brothers that were apparently affected by PHP-Ib [61], but other than this single report there is no evidence that PHP-Ib is caused by mutations in Gsα-coding *GNAS* exons.

As shown by a study in 1998 [62], PTH resistance in PHP-Ib develops only after maternal inheritance of the genetic defect, i.e. the mode of inheritance of the hormone resistance in PHP-Ib is similar to that in PHP-Ia. The same study has identified, through a genome-wide linkage analysis using four large kindreds with autosomal dominant PHP-Ib (AD-PHP-Ib), a genetic locus on chromosome 20q that included *GNAS* at its telomeric boundary, thus suggesting that the cause of PHP-Ib could be mutations within or near *GNAS*. In addition to Gsα, *GNAS* gives rise to several different transcripts that use promoters and first exons that are located upstream of the 13 exons that encode Gsα [63–66] (fig. 1). There is also a transcript formed in the opposite direction, i.e. *GNAS* antisense transcript [67, 68]. These relatively recently described transcripts show exclusively monoallelic expression, unlike Gsα which is biallelic in most tissues, as explained above. The transcript encoding a chromogranin-like neuroendocrine secretory protein (NESP55) is expressed maternally, while extra-large αs (XLαs), A/B (also known as 1A or 1′), and antisense transcripts are expressed

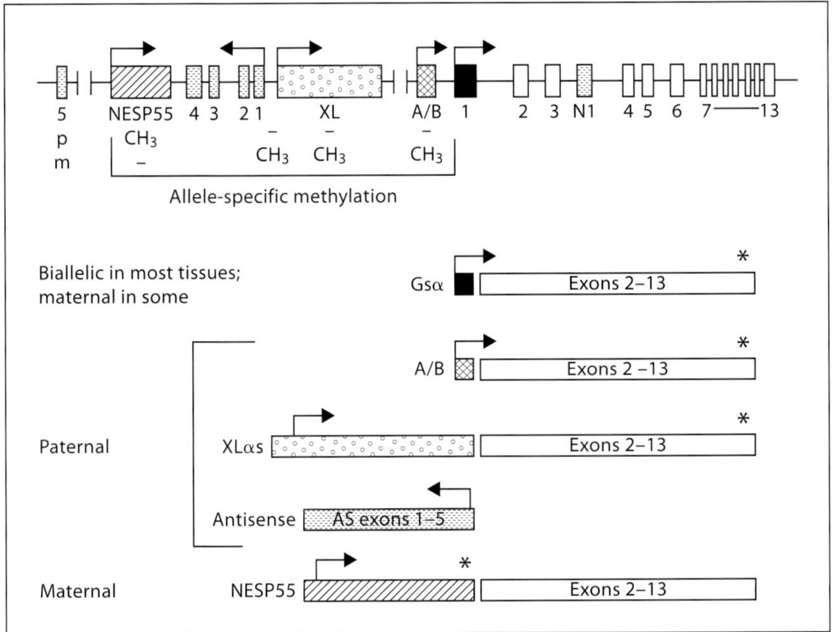

Fig. 1. The *GNAS* complex locus and its products. The gene structure is depicted above, with boxes and interconnecting lines indicating exons and introns, respectively. Arrows indicate the direction of transcription. Allele-specific methylation (CH_3) is indicated below the gene depiction. p = Paternal; m = maternal. The different *GNAS* products are depicted by rectangles, specifying the individual first exons in different shading for Gsα, A/B, XLαs, and NESP55. The asterisk indicates the location of the termination codon. The parental origin of each product is indicated on the left. Note that Gsα is predominantly maternal in several different tissues including the renal proximal tubule, thyroid, pituitary, gonads, and certain parts of the brain.

paternally [32, 33, 35, 68, 69]. Consistent with this parent-of-origin specific expression, the promoters of these transcripts, unlike the promoter of Gsα, are differentially methylated, with the methylation being on the silenced allele (fig. 1).

A study by Liu et al. [70] showed in 2000 that patients with PHP-Ib have methylation changes in the *GNAS* locus. Some patients display epigenetic alterations in multiple regions within *GNAS*, but the most consistent defect is a loss of methylation at the A/B differentially methylated region (DMR). The latter epigenetic defect, which occurs on the maternal allele, is thought to silence the downstream Gsα promoter *in cis* but only in those tissues in which Gsα is already silenced from the paternal allele, such as the renal proximal tubule, thus leading to a severe reduction in Gsα expression levels. Subsequent genetic studies by using additional AD-PHP-Ib kindreds have led to the identification of a recurrent 3-kb deletion located more than 200 kb upstream of the *GNAS* locus [71]. The deleted region is flanked by two 391-bp direct repeats, and in genomic DNA of patients carrying the 3-kb deletion, only one of these direct repeats is present, suggesting that these repeats contribute to the formation of the deletion through a mechanism involving homologous recombination. PHP-Ib and the isolated loss of A/B methylation are present only in those individuals who inherited the deletion from a female obligate carrier, whereas there is no phenotype in those who inherited the same deletion paternally. This is consistent with the imprinted mode of inheritance for this disease. Interestingly, the 3-kb deletion removes exons 4–6 of another gene, *STX16*, which encodes syntaxin 16. In a single unrelated AD-PHP-Ib kindred, a deletion of 4.4 kb removing *STX16* exons 2–4 has subsequently been identified [72]. Similar to the AD-PHP-Ib kindreds in whom the genetic defect is the 3-kb deletion, patients carrying the 4.4-kb deletion show a loss of methylation only at the A/B DMR. *STX16* does not appear to be imprinted [72], and it is unlikely that the loss of the maternal *STX16* allele is the cause of PTH resistance and the loss of methylation at the A/B DMR. Instead, it appears likely that the deletion disrupts a *cis*-acting element that regulates the establishment or maintenance of methylation on the maternal A/B region. However, this hypothesis has yet to be proven as targeted removal of the region equivalent to the 3-kb *STX16* deletion in mice does not lead to any phenotype [73].

Few AD-PHP-Ib kindreds show methylation alterations at all *GNAS* DMRs, including loss of methylation at the promoters and first exons of A/B, XLαs, and antisense transcripts and a gain of methylation at the promoter and first exon of NESP55. In two such kindreds, maternally inherited deletions that remove the entire DMR comprising exon NESP55 and exons 3 and 4 of the *GNAS* antisense transcript have been identified [74]. A mouse model in which the entire NESP55 DMR is deleted has been generated, and these mice show broad methylation defects of *GNAS* that are similar to those observed in the patients, as well as hypocalcemia, hyperphosphatemia, and elevated serum PTH [75, 76]. Another deletion has subsequently been discovered in an unrelated AD-PHP-Ib kindred in whom affected individuals showed broad *GNAS* methylation defects. The latter deletion removed exons 3 and 4 of the antisense transcript but not the exon encoding NESP55 [77]. It is therefore likely that the region immediately downstream of NESP55 includes another *cis*-acting regulatory element necessary for the establishment or the maintenance of all the maternal *GNAS* imprint marks. However, a study by Chotalia et al. [78] has shown that transcription from an oocyte-specific Nesp55 promoter is required for the establishment of these imprint marks in mice, making it possible that the disruption of the NESP55 transcript, rather than the removal of this putative *cis*-acting element, is the cause of PHP-Ib in these AD-PHP-Ib kindreds with broad *GNAS* methylation changes. Recently, a 19-kb deletion extending from the region upstream of the NESP55 DMR to antisense exon 4 has been discovered in an unrelated AD-PHP-Ib kindred [79]. Interestingly, the patients carrying this deletion on the maternal allele displayed a loss of methylation at exon A/B without imprinting defects at other *GNAS* DMRs, indicating that some deletions involving the NESP55 DMR can be associated with isolated loss of exon A/B imprinting [79]. The latter finding is in fact consistent with those obtained in the study by Chotalia et al. [78], in which the truncation of maternal transcripts from the Nesp55 promoter led to an isolated loss of exon A/B (termed 1A in mice) methylation in a significant portion of the offspring.

Each deletion causing AD-PHP-Ib is associated with *GNAS* methylation changes only when located on the maternal allele, with the exception of the deletion removing only exons 3 and 4 of the *GNAS* antisense transcript [77]. While the maternal inheritance of the latter deletion causes PTH resistance and broad *GNAS* methylation changes on the maternal allele, it has been shown that the unaffected carriers, who inherited the deletion paternally, also show methylation changes, including an incomplete loss of NESP55 methylation and an incomplete gain of A/B methylation [77]. The latter epigenetic change might predict that the unaffected carriers have increased PTH sensitivity in the renal proximal tubule, as a study in mice has shown that partial gain of A/B methylation increases Gsα levels in tissues in which this protein is normally silenced from the paternal allele [80]. Consistent with this prediction, one of the three unaffected carriers in this AD-PHP-Ib kindred had reduced serum PTH and elevated 1,25 dihydroxy vitamin D levels [77].

Sporadic PHP-Ib cases also show *GNAS* methylation defects, but these defects are present typically at the A/B DMR and at least one additional *GNAS* DMR [70, 81–83]. In those sporadic cases in whom the *GNAS* methylation defects involve all the *GNAS* DMRs, paternal UPD involving chromosome 20q has been documented as the cause of the disease [59, 84–86]. The cause of these epigenetic alterations in many other cases remains currently unknown. Given that the methylation defects in the sporadic PHP-Ib cases are quite similar to those observed in AD-PHP-Ib kindreds who carry deletions affecting the NESP55 DMR, it is likely that some of the sporadic PHP-Ib cases carry mutations in this region, which could occur de novo either on the maternal allele of the patient or on the paternal allele of the patient's mother. However, some sporadic PHP-Ib patients share the maternal *GNAS* haplotype with their unaffected siblings, and some others transmit the maternal allele in this region to their unaffected offspring, thus arguing against mutations within *GNAS* as the cause of the disease [87]. It is possible that the cause of these methylation defects in sporadic PHP-Ib cases is disruption of a putative *trans*-acting factor necessary for the establishment or the maintenance of the methylation imprints on the maternal *GNAS* allele. Potential candidates for this putative factor could be *NLRP7* and *ZFP57*, mutations of which cause certain types of hydatidiform mole and transient neonatal diabetes, respectively, and disrupt the imprinting of multiple genes including, in some cases, the *GNAS* locus [88–90]. However, disease-causing mutations in these two genes could not be identified as the cause of PHP-Ib in 3 independent cases in whom the *GNAS* locus was genetically excluded [87].

Some recent findings obtained by analyzing various patients with PTH resistance have revealed that the clinical and genetic features of PHP-Ia and PHP-Ib may overlap. In a number of patients who have AHO features and PTH resistance, coding mutations in Gsα have been excluded, but instead, epigenetic alterations within *GNAS* have been demonstrated [91–94]. These findings may suggest that these AHO features reflect the silencing of the paternal Gsα allele in tissues that are previously unrecognized. Consistent with this interpretation, recent studies have indeed shown that the maternal Gsα expression is higher than the paternal expression in erythrocytes and certain other blood cells, as well as mammary adipose tissue and heart [95, 96]. However, in some cases it is possible that the AHO features result from large maternal deletions of *GNAS* that cause both Gsα haploinsufficiency and an apparent loss of imprinting at this locus. In fact, a maternal 30-kb deletion that extends from the A/B region to *GNAS* exon 5 has been revealed as the cause of these findings in a single case [97]. Consistent with the presence of this deletion, the Gsα bioactivity in the erythrocytes derived from the latter patient was significantly reduced [91], and therefore, this valuable test or other investigations that would rule out a similar *GNAS* deletion, such as analysis of polymorphisms, should be performed before concluding that AHO features observed in a patient with loss of *GNAS* imprinting is truly due to the latter defect.

PHP type II is less well characterized than PHP type I [3]. Since urinary cAMP excretion in response to exogenous PTH administration is not blunted in patients with PHP type II, the genetic defect leading to this PHP type is predicted to lie downstream of Gsα and adenylyl cyclase, the enzyme catalyzing the synthesis of cAMP. Recently, 3 patients have been described who could be classified as having PHP type II based on the presence of PTH and other hormone resistance with an unimpaired urinary cAMP excretion in response to recombinant PTH infusion [98]. No PTH-induced urinary phosphate excretion was observed in these patients. Moreover, PTH-induced inhibition of urinary fractional calcium excretion was impaired, consistent with PTH resistance. Note, however, that this defect in the action of PTH on urinary calcium excretion is not predicted to be present in PHP-Ia and PHP-Ib patients, because Gsα expression is not paternally silenced in the distal nephron [26]. In addition to multi-hormone resistance with unimpaired PTH-induced urinary cAMP excretion, the recently described patients had skeletal dysplasia termed acrodysostosis, which resemble, but are more severe than, the skeletal abnormalities in AHO including brachydactyly and short stature [98]. Genetic analysis of these patients revealed a heterozygous non-sense mutation of the gene encoding cAMP-dependent protein kinase (PKA) type Iα regulatory subunit (PRKAR1A). The mutant PRKAR1A protein, which lacks the last 14 C-terminal amino acids, is unable to respond to cAMP and, thus, prevents the activation of PKA. The hormone resistance profile in these patients may perhaps reflect the cell-specific expression profiles of PRKAR1A and other PKA subunits. Recent studies have identified additional PRKAR1A mutations in patients with similar clinical findings [99, 100].

In summary, PHP refers to a group of related disorders characterized primarily by end-organ resistance to PTH. The genetic defects responsible for the different forms of PHP disrupt the mechanisms leading to the formation of cAMP or the activation of downstream effectors. PHP type I is caused by inactivating mutations within Gsα-coding *GNAS* exons (PHP-Ia, PPHP, and, in some cases, PHP-Ic) or mutations altering the imprinting of *GNAS* and, thereby, the expression of Gsα in certain tissues (PHP-Ib). PHP type II is caused by mutations altering the activity of PRKAR1A. Discovery of novel mutations underlying these disorders will be important for gaining a better understanding of the mechanisms underlying PTH resistance and for providing genetic counseling to patients and their families.

Acknowledgement

Studies performed in the author's lab have been funded by grants from the National Institutes of Diabetes and Digestive and Kidney Diseases, the March of Dimes Foundation, and the Milton Fund.

References

1 Albright F, Burnett CH, Smith PH, Parson W: Pseudohypoparathyroidism – an example of 'Seabright-Bantam syndrome'. Endocrinology 1942;30:922–932.

2 Chase LR, Melson GL, Aurbach GD: Pseudohypoparathyroidism: defective excretion of 3′,5′-AMP in response to parathyroid hormone. J Clin Invest 1969;48:1832–1844.

3 Drezner M, Neelon FA, Lebovitz HE: Pseudohypoparathyroidism type II: a possible defect in the reception of the cyclic AMP signal. N Engl J Med 1973;289:1056–1060.

4 Levine MA, Downs RW Jr, Moses AM, Breslau NA, Marx SJ, Lasker RD, Rizzoli RE, Aurbach GD, Spiegel AM: Resistance to multiple hormones in patients with pseudohypoparathyroidism. Association with deficient activity of guanine nucleotide regulatory protein. Am J Med 1983;74:545–556.

5 Mallet E, Carayon P, Amr S, Brunelle P, Ducastelle T, Basuyau JP, de Menibus CH: Coupling defect of thyrotropin receptor and adenylate cyclase in a pseudohypoparathyroid patient. J Clin Endocrinol Metab 1982;54:1028–1032.

6 Wolfsdorf JI, Rosenfield RL, Fang VS, Kobayashi R, Razdan AK, Kim MH: Partial gonadotrophin-resistance in pseudohypoparathyroidism. Acta Endocrinol (Copenh) 1978;88:321–328.

7 Stirling HF, Barr DGD, Kelnar CJH: Familial growth hormone releasing factor deficiency in pseudohypoparathyroidism. Arch Dis Child 1991; 66:533–535.

8 Namnoum AB, Merriam GR, Moses AM, Levine MA: Reproductive dysfunction in women with Albright's hereditary osteodystrophy. J Clin Endocrinol Metab 1998;83:824–829.

9 Mantovani G, Maghnie M, Weber G, De Menis E, Brunelli V, Cappa M, Loli P, Beck-Peccoz P, Spada A: Growth hormone-releasing hormone resistance in pseudohypoparathyroidism type Ia: new evidence for imprinting of the Gs alpha gene. J Clin Endocrinol Metab 2003;88:4070–4074.

10 Germain-Lee EL, Groman J, Crane JL, Jan de Beur SM, Levine MA: Growth hormone deficiency in pseudohypoparathyroidism type 1a: another manifestation of multihormone resistance. J Clin Endocrinol Metab 2003;88:4059–4069.

11 Weinstein LS, Gejman PV, Friedman E, Kadowaki T, Collins RM, Gershon ES, Spiegel AM: Mutations of the Gs alpha-subunit gene in Albright hereditary osteodystrophy detected by denaturing gradient gel electrophoresis. Proc Natl Acad Sci USA 1990;87: 8287–8290.

12 Patten JL, Johns DR, Valle D, Eil C, Gruppuso PA, Steele G, Smallwood PM, Levine MA: Mutation in the gene encoding the stimulatory G protein of adenylate cyclase in Albright's hereditary osteodystrophy. N Engl J Med 1990;322:1412–1419.

13 Kozasa T, Itoh H, Tsukamoto T, Kaziro Y: Isolation and characterization of the human Gsα gene. Proc Natl Acad Sci USA 1988;85:2081–2085.

14 Gejman PV, Weinstein LS, Martinez M, Spiegel AM, Cao Q, Hsieh WT, Hoehe MR, Gershon ES: Genetic mapping of the Gs-alpha subunit gene (GNAS1) to the distal long arm of chromosome 20 using a polymorphism detected by denaturing gradient gel electrophoresis. Genomics 1991;9:782–783.

15 Rao VV, Schnittger S, Hansmann I: G protein Gs alpha (GNAS 1), the probable candidate gene for Albright hereditary osteodystrophy, is assigned to human chromosome 20q12-q13.2. Genomics 1991; 10:257–261.

16 Levine MA, Modi WS, O'Brien SJ: Mapping of the gene encoding the alpha subunit of the stimulatory G protein of adenylyl cyclase (GNAS1) to 20q13.2 → q13.3 in human by in situ hybridization. Genomics 1991;11:478–479.
17 Gilman AG: G proteins: Transducers of receptor-generated signals. Ann Rev Biochem 1987;56:615–649.
18 Spiegel AM: Introduction to G-protein-coupled signal transduction and human disease. In: AM Spiegel (ed), G Proteins, Receptors, and Disease. Humana Press, Totowa, 1998, pp 1–21.
19 Cabrera-Vera TM, Vanhauwe J, Thomas TO, Medkova M, Preininger A, Mazzoni MR, Hamm HE: Insights into G protein structure, function, and regulation. Endocr Rev 2003;24:765–781.
20 Moses AM, Weinstock RS, Levine MA, Breslau NA: Evidence for normal antidiuretic responses to endogenous and exogenous arginine vasopressin in patients with guanine nucleotide-binding stimulatory protein-deficient pseudohypoparathyroidism. J Clin Endocrinol Metab 1986;62:221–224.
21 Weinstein LS: Albright hereditary osteodystrophy, pseudohypoparathyroidism, and G_s deficiency. In: AM Spiegel (ed), G Proteins, Receptors, and Disease. Humana Press, Totowa, 1998, pp. 23–56.
22 Levine MA: Pseudohypoparathyroidism: from bedside to bench and back. J Bone Miner Res 1999;14: 1255–1260.
23 Albright F, Forbes AP, Henneman PH: Pseudo-pseudohypoparathyroidism. Trans Assoc Am Physicians 1952;65:337–350.
24 Davies AJ, Hughes HE: Imprinting in Albright's hereditary osteodystrophy. J Med Genet 1993;30: 101–103.
25 Yu S, Yu D, Lee E, Eckhaus M, Lee R, Corria Z, Accili D, Westphal H, Weinstein LS: Variable and tissue-specific hormone resistance in heterotrimeric G_s protein α-subunit ($G_s\alpha$) knockout mice is due to tissue-specific imprinting of the $G_s\alpha$ gene. Proc Natl Acad Sci USA 1998;95:8715–8720.
26 Weinstein LS, Yu S, Ecelbarger CA: Variable imprinting of the heterotrimeric G protein G(s) alpha-subunit within different segments of the nephron. Am J Physiol Renal Physiol 2000;278: F507–F514.
27 Liu J, Erlichman B, Weinstein LS: The stimulatory G protein α-subunit Gsα is imprinted in human thyroid glands: implications for thyroid function in pseudohypoparathyroidism types 1A and 1B. J Clin Endocrinol Metabol 2003;88:4336–4341.
28 Mantovani G, Ballare E, Giammona E, Beck-Peccoz P, Spada A: The Gsalpha gene: predominant maternal origin of transcription in human thyroid gland and gonads. J Clin Endocrinol Metab 2002;87: 4736–4740.
29 Germain-Lee EL, Ding CL, Deng Z, Crane JL, Saji M, Ringel MD, Levine MA: Paternal imprinting of Galpha(s) in the human thyroid as the basis of TSH resistance in pseudohypoparathyroidism type 1a. Biochem Biophys Res Commun 2002;296:67–72.
30 Hayward B, Barlier A, Korbonits M, Grossman A, Jacquet P, Enjalbert A, Bonthron D: Imprinting of the G(s)alpha gene GNAS1 in the pathogenesis of acromegaly. J Clin Invest 2001;107:R31–R36.
31 Chen M, Wang J, Dickerson KE, Kelleher J, Xie T, Gupta D, Lai EW, Pacak K, Gavrilova O, Weinstein LS: Central nervous system imprinting of the G protein G(s)alpha and its role in metabolic regulation. Cell Metab 2009;9:548–555.
32 Hayward B, Kamiya M, Strain L, Moran V, Campbell R, Hayashizaki Y, Bonthon DT: The human GNAS1 gene is imprinted and encodes distinct paternally and biallelically expressed G proteins. Proc Natl Acad Sci USA 1998;95:10038–10043.
33 Hayward BE, Moran V, Strain L, Bonthron DT: Bidirectional imprinting of a single gene: GNAS1 encodes maternally, paternally, and biallelically derived proteins. Proc Natl Acad Sci USA 1998; 95:15475–15480.
34 Campbell R, Gosden CM, Bonthron DT: Parental origin of transcription from the human GNAS1 gene. J Med Genet 1994;31:607–614.
35 Peters J, Wroe SF, Wells CA, Miller HJ, Bodle D, Beechey CV, Williamson CM, Kelsey G: A cluster of oppositely imprinted transcripts at the Gnas locus in the distal imprinting region of mouse chromosome 2. Proc Natl Acad Sci USA 1999;96:3830–3835.
36 Mantovani G, Bondioni S, Locatelli M, Pedroni C, Lania AG, Ferrante E, Filopanti M, Beck-Peccoz P, Spada A: Biallelic expression of the Gsalpha gene in human bone and adipose tissue. J Clin Endocrinol Metab 2004;89:6316–6319.
37 Bastepe M, Weinstein LS, Ogata N, Kawaguchi H, Jüppner H, Kronenberg HM, Chung UI: Stimulatory G protein directly regulates hypertrophic differentiation of growth plate cartilage in vivo. Proc Natl Acad Sci USA 2004;101:14794–14799.
38 Long DN, McGuire S, Levine MA, Weinstein LS, Germain-Lee EL: Body mass index differences in pseudohypoparathyroidism type 1a versus pseudopseudohypoparathyroidism may implicate paternal imprinting of Galpha(s) in the development of human obesity. J Clin Endocrinol Metab 2007;92: 1073–1079.

39 Mouallem M, Shaharabany M, Weintrob N, Shalitin S, Nagelberg N, Shapira H, Zadik Z, Farfel Z: Cognitive impairment is prevalent in pseudohypoparathyroidism type Ia, but not in pseudopseudohypoparathyroidism: possible cerebral imprinting of Gsalpha. Clin Endocrinol (Oxf) 2008;68:233–239.
40 Levine MA, Jap TS, Mauseth RS, Downs J, Spiegel AM: Activity of the stimulatory guanine nucleotide-binding protein is reduced in erythrocytes from patients with pseudohypoparathyroidism and pseudohypoparathyroidism: biochemical, endocrine, and genetic analysis of Albright's hereditary osteodystrophy in six kindreds. J Clin Endocrinol Metab 1986;62:497–502.
41 Miric A, Vechio JD, Levine MA: Heterogeneous mutations in the gene encoding the alpha-subunit of the stimulatory G protein of adenylyl cyclase in Albright hereditary osteodystrophy. J Clin Endocrinol Metab 1993;76:1560–1568.
42 Farfel Z, Bourne HR: Deficient activity of receptor-cyclase coupling protein in platelets of patients with pseudohypoparathyroidism. J Clin Endocrinol Metab 1980;51:1202–1204.
43 Farfel Z, Brothers VM, Brickman AS, Conte F, Neer R, Bourne HR: Pseudohypoparathyroidism: inheritance of deficient receptor-cyclase coupling activity. Proc Natl Acad Sci USA1981;78:3098–3102.
44 Bourne HR, Kaslow HR, Brickman AS, Farfel Z: Fibroblast defect in pseudohypoparathyroidism, type I: reduced activity of receptor-cyclase coupling protein. J Clin Endocrinol Metab 1981;53:636–640.
45 Spiegel AM, Levine MA, Aurbach GD, Downs RW, Jr, Marx SJ, Lasker RD, Moses AM, Breslau NA: Deficiency of hormone receptor-adenylate cyclase coupling protein: basis for hormone resistance in pseudohypoparathyroidism. Am J Physiol 1982;243: E37–E42.
46 Motulsky HJ, Hughes RJ, Brickman AS, Farfel Z, Bourne HR, Insel PA: Platelets of pseudohypoparathyroid patients: evidence that distinct receptor-cyclase coupling proteins mediate stimulation and inhibition of adenylate cyclase. Proc Natl Acad Sci USA 1982;79:4193–4197.
47 Farfel Z, Abood ME, Brickman AS, Bourne HR: Deficient activity of receptor-cyclase coupling protein is transformed lymphoblasts of patients with pseudohypoparathyroidism, type I. J Clin Endocrinol Metab 1982;55:113–117.
48 Levine MA, Eil C, Downs RW Jr, Spiegel AM: Deficient guanine nucleotide regulatory unit activity in cultured fibroblast membranes from patients with pseudohypoparathyroidism type I. A cause of impaired synthesis of 3′,5′-cyclic AMP by intact and broken cells. J Clin Invest 1983;72:316–324.
49 Levine MA, Ahn TG, Klupt SF, Kaufman KD, Smallwood PM, Bourne HR, Sullivan KA, Van Dop C: Genetic deficiency of the alpha subunit of the guanine nucleotide-binding protein Gs as the molecular basis for Albright hereditary osteodystrophy. Proc Natl Acad Sci USA 1988;85:617–621.
50 Patten JL, Levine MA: Immunochemical analysis of the α-subunit of the stimulatory G-protein of adenylyl cyclase in patients with Albright's hereditary osteodystrophy. J Clin Endocrinol Metab 1990;71: 1208–1214.
51 Carter A, Bardin C, Collins R, Simons C, Bray P, Spiegel A: Reduced expression of multiple forms of the ααsubunit of the stimulatory GTP-binding protein in pseudohypoparathyroidism type Ia. Proc Natl Acad Sci USA 1987;84:7266–7269.
52 Levine MA, Downs RW Jr, Singer M, Marx SJ, Aurbach GD, Spiegel AM: Deficient activity of guanine nucleotide regulatory protein in erythrocytes from patients with pseudohypoparathyroidism. Biochem Biophys Res Commun 1980;94:1319–1324.
53 Linglart A, Carel JC, Garabedian M, Le T, Mallet E, Kottler ML: GNAS1 lesions in pseudohypoparathyroidism Ia and Ic: genotype phenotype relationship and evidence of the maternal transmission of the hormonal resistance. J Clin Endocrinol Metab 2002; 87:189–197.
54 Thiele S, de Sanctis L, Werner R, Grotzinger J, Aydin C, Juppner H, Bastepe M, Hiort O: Functional characterization of GNAS mutations found in patients with pseudohypoparathyroidism type Ic defines a new subgroup of pseudohypoparathyroidism affecting selectively Gsalpha-receptor interaction. Hum Mutat 2011;32:653–660.
55 Linglart A, Mahon MJ, Kerachian MA, Berlach DM, Hendy GN, Jüppner H, Bastepe M: Coding GNAS mutations leading to hormone resistance impair in vitro agonist- and cholera toxin-induced adenosine cyclic 3′,5′-monophosphate formation mediated by human XLαs. Endocrinology 2006; 147:2253–2262.
56 Peterman MG, Garvey JL: Pseudohypoparathyroidism; case report. Pediatrics 1949;4:790.
57 Reynolds TB, Jacobson G, Edmondson HA, Martin HE, Nelson CH: Pseudohypoparathyroidism: report of a case showing bony demineralization. J Clin Endocrinol Metab 1952;12:560.
58 Bastepe M, Pincus JE, Sugimoto T, Tojo K, Kanatani M, Azuma Y, Kruse K, Rosenbloom AL, Koshiyama H, Jüppner H: Positional dissociation between the genetic mutation responsible for pseudohypoparathyroidism type Ib and the associated methylation defect at exon A/B: evidence for a long-range regulatory element within the imprinted *GNAS1* locus. Hum Mol Genet 2001;10:1231–1241.

59 Bastepe M, Lane AH, Jüppner H: Paternal uniparental isodisomy of chromosome 20q (patUPD20q) – and the resulting changes in *GNAS1* methylation – as a plausible cause of pseudohypoparathyroidism. Am J Hum Genet 2001;68:1283–1289.
60 Mantovani G, Bondioni S, Linglart A, Maghnie M, Cisternino M, Corbetta S, Lania AG, Beck-Peccoz P, Spada A: Genetic analysis and evaluation of resistance to thyrotropin and growth hormone-releasing hormone in pseudohypoparathyroidism type Ib. J Clin Endocrinol Metab 2007;92:3738–3742.
61 Wu WI, Schwindinger WF, Aparicio LF, Levine MA: Selective resistance to parathyroid hormone caused by a novel uncoupling mutation in the carboxyl terminus of Gαs: a cause of pseudohypoparathyroidism type Ib. J Biol Chem 2001;276:165–171.
62 Jüppner H, Schipani E, Bastepe M, Cole DEC, Lawson ML, Mannstadt M, Hendy GN, Plotkin H, Koshiyama H, Koh T, Crawford JD, Olsen BR, Vikkula M: The gene responsible for pseudohypoparathyroidism type Ib is paternally imprinted and maps in four unrelated kindreds to chromosome 20q13.3. Proc Natl Acad Sci USA 1998;95:11798–11803.
63 Ischia R, Lovisetti-Scamihorn P, Hogue-Angeletti R, Wolkersdorfer M, Winkler H, Fischer-Colbrie R: Molecular cloning and characterization of NESP55, a novel chromogranin-like precursor of a peptide with 5-HT1B receptor antagonist activity. J Biol Chem 1997;272:11657–11662.
64 Kehlenbach RH, Matthey J, Huttner WB: XLαs is a new type of G protein. Nature 1994;372:804–809, erratum Nature 1995;375:253.
65 Swaroop A, Agarwal N, Gruen JR, Bick D, Weissman SM: Differential expression of novel Gs alpha signal transduction protein cDNA species. Nucleic Acids Res 1991;19:4725–4729.
66 Ishikawa Y, Bianchi C, Nadal-Ginard B, Homcy CJ: Alternative promoter and 5′ exon generate a novel $G_s\alpha$ mRNA. J Biol Chem 1990;265:8458–8462.
67 Hayward B, Bonthron D: An imprinted antisense transcript at the human GNAS1 locus. Hum Mol Genet 2000;9:835–841.
68 Wroe SF, Kelsey G, Skinner JA, Bodle D, Ball ST, Beechey CV, Peters J, Williamson CM: An imprinted transcript, antisense to Nesp, adds complexity to the cluster of imprinted genes at the mouse Gnas locus. Proc Natl Acad Sci USA 2000;97:3342–3346.
69 Liu J, Yu S, Litman D, Chen W, Weinstein L: Identification of a methylation imprint mark within the mouse Gnas locus. Mol Cell Biol 2000;20:5808–5817.
70 Liu J, Litman D, Rosenberg M, Yu S, Biesecker L, Weinstein L: A GNAS1 imprinting defect in pseudohypoparathyroidism type IB. J Clin Invest 2000;106:1167–1174.
71 Bastepe M, Fröhlich LF, Hendy GN, Indridason OS, Josse RG, Koshiyama H, Körkkö J, Nakamoto JM, Rosenbloom AL, Slyper AH, Sugimoto T, Tsatsoulis A, Crawford JD, Jüppner H: Autosomal dominant pseudohypoparathyroidism type Ib is associated with a heterozygous microdeletion that likely disrupts a putative imprinting control element of GNAS. J Clin Invest 2003;112:1255–1263.
72 Linglart A, Gensure RC, Olney RC, Jüppner H, Bastepe M: A Novel STX16 deletion in autosomal dominant pseudohypoparathyroidism type Ib redefines the boundaries of a cis-acting imprinting control element of GNAS. Am J Hum Genet 2005;76:804–814.
73 Fröhlich LF, Bastepe M, Ozturk D, Abu-Zahra H, Jüppner H: Lack of Gnas epigenetic changes and pseudohypoparathyroidism type Ib in mice with targeted disruption of syntaxin-16. Endocrinology 2007;148:2925–2935.
74 Bastepe M, Fröhlich LF, Linglart A, Abu-zahra HS, Tojo K, Ward LM, Jüppner H: Deletion of the NESP55 differentially methylated region causes loss of maternal GNAS imprints and pseudohypoparathyroidism type-Ib. Nat Genet 2005;37:25–37.
75 Fröhlich LF, Mrakovcic M, Steinborn R, Chung UI, Bastepe M, Juppner H: Targeted deletion of the Nesp55 DMR defines another Gnas imprinting control region and provides a mouse model of autosomal dominant PHP-Ib. Proc Natl Acad Sci USA 2010;107:9275–9280.
76 Fernandez-Rebollo E, Maeda A, Reyes M, Turan S, Frohlich LF, Plagge A, Kelsey G, Juppner H, Bastepe M: Loss of XLalphas (extra-large alphas) imprinting results in early postnatal hypoglycemia and lethality in a mouse model of pseudohypoparathyroidism Ib. Proc Natl Acad Sci USA 2012;109:6638–6643.
77 Chillambhi S, Turan S, Hwang DY, Chen HC, Juppner H, Bastepe M: Deletion of the noncoding GNAS antisense transcript causes pseudohypoparathyroidism type Ib and biparental defects of GNAS methylation in cis. J Clin Endocrinol Metab 2010;95:3993–4002.
78 Chotalia M, Smallwood SA, Ruf N, Dawson C, Lucifero D, Frontera M, James K, Dean W, Kelsey G: Transcription is required for establishment of germline methylation marks at imprinted genes. Genes Dev 2009;23:105–117.

79 Richard N, Abeguile G, Coudray N, Mittre H, Gruchy N, Andrieux J, Cathebras P, Kottler ML: A new deletion ablating NESP55 causes loss of maternal imprint of A/B GNAS and autosomal dominant pseudohypoparathyroidism type Ib. J Clin Endocrinol Metab 2012;97:E863–E867.
80 Williamson CM, Turner MD, Ball ST, Nottingham WT, Glenister P, Fray M, Tymowska-Lalanne Z, Plagge A, Powles-Glover N, Kelsey G, Maconochie M, Peters J: Identification of an imprinting control region affecting the expression of all transcripts in the Gnas cluster. Nat Genet 2006;38:350–355.
81 Linglart A, Bastepe M, Jüppner H: Similar clinical and laboratory findings in patients with symptomatic autosomal dominant and sporadic pseudohypoparathyroidism type Ib despite different epigenetic changes at the GNAS locus. Clin Endocrinol (Oxf) 2007;67:822–831.
82 Maupetit-Mehouas S, Mariot V, Reynes C, Bertrand G, Feillet F, Carel JC, Simon D, Bihan H, Gajdos V, Devouge E, Shenoy S, Agbo-Kpati P, Ronan A, Naud-Saudreau C, Lienhardt A, Silve C, Linglart A: Quantification of the methylation at the GNAS locus identifies subtypes of sporadic pseudohypoparathyroidism type Ib. J Med Genet 2011;48:55–63.
83 Liu J, Nealon JG, Weinstein LS: Distinct patterns of abnormal GNAS imprinting in familial and sporadic pseudohypoparathyroidism type IB. Hum Mol Genet 2005;14:95–102.
84 Bastepe M, Altug-Teber O, Agarwal C, Oberfield SE, Bonin M, Jüppner H: Paternal uniparental isodisomy of the entire chromosome 20 as a molecular cause of pseudohypoparathyroidism type Ib (PHP-Ib). Bone 2011;48:659–662.
85 Lecumberri B, Fernandez-Rebollo E, Sentchordi L, Saavedra P, Bernal-Chico A, Pallardo LF, Jimenez Bustos JM, Castano L, De Santiago M, Hiort O, Perez de Nanclares G, Bastepe M: Coexistence of two different pseudohypoparathyroidism subtypes (Ia and Ib) in the same kindred with independent Gsα coding mutations and GNAS imprinting defects. J Med Genet 2010;47:276–280.
86 Fernandez-Rebollo E, Lecumberri B, Garin I, Arroyo J, Bernal-Chico A, Goni F, Orduna R, Castano L, Perez de Nanclares G: New mechanisms involved in paternal 20q disomy associated with pseudohypoparathyroidism. Eur J Endocrinol 2010;163:953–962.
87 Fernandez-Rebollo E, Perez de Nanclares G, Lecumberri B, Turan S, Anda E, Perez-Nanclares G, Feig D, Nik-Zainal S, Bastepe M, Juppner H: Exclusion of the GNAS locus in PHP-Ib patients with broad GNAS methylation changes: evidence for an autosomal recessive form of PHP-Ib? J Bone Miner Res 2011;26:1854–1863.
88 Judson H, Hayward BE, Sheridan E, Bonthron DT: A global disorder of imprinting in the human female germ line. Nature 2002;416:539–542.
89 Murdoch S, Djuric U, Mazhar B, Seoud M, Khan R, Kuick R, Bagga R, Kircheisen R, Ao A, Ratti B, Hanash S, Rouleau GA, Slim R: Mutations in NALP7 cause recurrent hydatidiform moles and reproductive wastage in humans. Nat Genet 2006;38:300–302.
90 Mackay DJ, Callaway JL, Marks SM, White HE, Acerini CL, Boonen SE, Dayanikli P, Firth HV, Goodship JA, Haemers AP, Hahnemann JM, Kordonouri O, Masoud AF, Oestergaard E, Storr J, Ellard S, Hattersley AT, Robinson DO, Temple IK: Hypomethylation of multiple imprinted loci in individuals with transient neonatal diabetes is associated with mutations in ZFP57. Nat Genet 2008;40:949–951.
91 de Nanclares GP, Fernandez-Rebollo E, Santin I, Garcia-Cuartero B, Gaztambide S, Menendez E, Morales MJ, Pombo M, Bilbao JR, Barros F, Zazo N, Ahrens W, Jüppner H, Hiort O, Castano L, Bastepe M: Epigenetic defects of GNAS in patients with pseudohypoparathyroidism and mild features of Albright's hereditary osteodystrophy. J Clin Endocrinol Metab 2007;92:2370–2373.
92 Mariot V, Maupetit-Mehouas S, Sinding C, Kottler ML, Linglart A: A maternal epimutation of GNAS leads to Albright osteodystrophy and parathyroid hormone resistance. J Clin Endocrinol Metab 2008;93:661–665.
93 Unluturk U, Harmanci A, Babaoglu M, Yasar U, Varli K, Bastepe M, Bayraktar M: Molecular diagnosis and clinical characterization of pseudohypoparathyroidism type-Ib in a patient with mild Albright's hereditary osteodystrophy-like features, epileptic seizures, and defective renal handling of uric acid. Am J Med Sci 2008;336:84–90.
94 Mantovani G, de Sanctis L, Barbieri AM, Elli FM, Bollati V, Vaira V, Labarile P, Bondioni S, Peverelli E, Lania AG, Beck-Peccoz P, Spada A: Pseudohypoparathyroidism and GNAS epigenetic defects: clinical evaluation of albright hereditary osteodystrophy and molecular analysis in 40 patients. J Clin Endocrinol Metab 2010;95:651–658.
95 Klenke S, Siffert W, Frey UH: A novel aspect of GNAS imprinting: higher maternal expression of Galphas in human lymphoblasts, peripheral blood mononuclear cells, mammary adipose tissue, and heart. Mol Cell Endocrinol 2011;341:63–70.

96 Zazo C, Thiele S, Martin C, Fernandez-Rebollo E, Martinez-Indart L, Werner R, Garin I, Hiort O, Perez de Nanclares G: Gsalpha activity is reduced in erythrocyte membranes of patients with pseudohypoparathyroidism due to epigenetic alterations at the GNAS locus. J Bone Miner Res 2011;26: 1864–1870.

97 Fernandez-Rebollo E, Garcia-Cuartero B, Garin I, Largo C, Martinez F, Garcia-Lacalle C, Castano L, Bastepe M, Perez de Nanclares G: Intragenic GNAS deletion involving exon A/B in pseudohypoparathyroidism type 1A resulting in an apparent loss of exon A/B methylation: potential for misdiagnosis of pseudohypoparathyroidism type 1B. J Clin Endocrinol Metab 2010;95:765–771.

98 Linglart A, Menguy C, Couvineau A, Auzan C, Gunes Y, Cancel M, Motte E, Pinto G, Chanson P, Bougneres P, Clauser E, Silve C: Recurrent PRKAR1A mutation in acrodysostosis with hormone resistance. N Engl J Med 2011;364:2218–2226.

99 Lee H, Graham JM Jr, Rimoin DL, Lachman RS, Krejci P, Tompson SW, Nelson SF, Krakow D, Cohn DH: Exome sequencing identifies PDE4D mutations in acrodysostosis. Am J Hum Genet 2012; 90:746–751.

100 Michot C, Le Goff C, Goldenberg A, Abhyankar A, Klein C, Kinning E, Guerrot AM, Flahaut P, Duncombe A, Baujat G, Lyonnet S, Thalassinos C, Nitschke P, Casanova JL, Le Merrer M, Munnich A, Cormier-Daire V: Exome sequencing identifies PDE4D mutations as another cause of acrodysostosis. Am J Hum Genet 2012;90:740–745.

Murat Bastepe, MD, PhD
Endocrine Unit, Massachusetts General Hospital
50 Blossom St. Thier 10
Boston, MA 02114 (USA)
E-Mail bastepe@helix.mgh.harvard.edu

Maghnie M, Loche S, Cappa M, Ghizzoni L, Lorini R (eds): Hormone Resistance and Hypersensitivity. From Genetics to Clinical Management. Endocr Dev. Basel, Karger, 2013, vol 24, pp 25–32 (DOI: 10.1159/000342496)

Gonadotropin Resistance

Ana Claudia Latronico · Ivo Jorge Prado Arnhold

Unidade de Endocrinologia do Desenvolvimento, Laboratório de Hormônios e Genética Molecular LIM/42, Hospital das Clínicas, Disciplina de Endocrinologia e Metabologia, Faculdade de Medicina da Universidade de São Paulo, São Paulo, Brasil

Abstract

Pituitary gonadotropins are essential for normal reproductive function. LH and FSH exert their effects by acting on G protein-coupled receptors. Pituitary LH and placental hCG share the same receptor (LHCGR). Homozygous or compound heterozygous inactivating mutations of LHCGR are associated with a phenotypic spectrum from female or ambiguous external genitalia due to Leydig cell hypoplasia to micropenis, hypergonadotropic hypogonadism and delayed puberty in genetic males. Testes size is slightly reduced, and testosterone levels are low in affected males. Interestingly, the clinical phenotypes are closely correlated with the severity of the mutation. In females, the phenotype is also variable and can range from primary amenorrhea to oligoamenorrhea, associated with constant infertility. Estradiol and progesterone levels remain in the early to mid-follicular phase, whereas the ovaries are normal or enlarged with cysts. In both sexes, LH levels are increased, whereas FSH is usually normal. Inactivating mutations of FSH receptor are associated with partial to complete premature ovarian failure in women and variable impairment of spermatogenesis and small testes in men. Mutations of the human gonadotropin receptors provide natural models for elucidating the differential effects of LH and FSH on the gonads.

Pituitary gonadotropic hormones have an essential role in the regulation of gonadal function. In genetic males, during sexual differentiation in the first trimester of embryogenesis, hCG stimulates testicular Leydig cells to produce androgen which induces virilization of the external genitalia. During the second and third trimesters of gestation, and again at puberty and during adulthood, LH stimulates the testes to promote penile growth and to induce the development and maintenance of secondary male sexual characteristics. FSH regulates Sertoli cell proliferation and differentiation, and participates in the regulation of spermatogenesis. In women, FSH induces follicular growth, and the subsequent LH surge induces ovulation. The secretion of gonadotropins is negatively controlled by gonadal sexual steroid hormones.

FSH and LH exert their actions by binding to specific membrane G protein-coupled receptors with large amino-terminal extracellular domains that contain a number of leucine-rich repeat motifs likely to be involved in protein-protein interactions, seven transmembrane helices and a C-terminal intracellular domain. The actions of LH and hCG are mediated by one membrane receptor, LHCG receptor, expressed in Leydig, mature granulosa cells and theca cells. The LHCG and FSH receptors activate various adenylyl cyclase isoenzymes, resulting in elevation of intracellular cAMP levels [1].

Human *LHCGR* and *FSHR* genes have been mapped to chromosome 2p21, and are composed of 11 and 10 exons, respectively. The final exons of both receptors encode the entire carboxyl terminal half of these receptors, including all seven transmembrane helices, the three interconnecting extracellular loops, the three interconnecting intracellular loops, and the cytoplasmic tail. A novel primate-specific exon (termed exon 6A) has recently been identified within intron 6 of the *LHCGR* gene [2]. This exon is not used by the wild-type full-length receptor. It displays composite characteristics of an internal/terminal exon and possesses stop codons triggering non-sense-mediated mRNA decay in *LHCGR*. When exon 6A is utilized, it results in a truncated LHCGR protein of only 209 amino acids that remains trapped intracellularly [2].

LH Resistance in Genetic Males

Several homozygous or compound-heterozygous inactivating mutations of the *LHCGR* have been described in 46,XY individuals with a rare form of disorder of sex development, termed Leydig cell hypoplasia, first described by Berthezene et al. [3]. These inactivating mutations in the LHCGR completely prevent LH and hCG signal transduction and thus testosterone production both pre- and postnatally in genetic males [4–16]. Leydig cell hypoplasia is an autosomal recessive disorder, characterized by a predominantly female external phenotype with a blind-ending vagina, primary amenorrhea, bilateral cryptorchidism and absent development of secondary sex characteristics at puberty [3–5]. Typically, these genetic male individuals have been raised as females, and have been diagnosed in their teens or early twenties when medical treatment was sought to determine their lack of breast development and primary amenorrhea [16, 17]. The undermasculization is associated with low testosterone levels and elevated LH levels, without abnormal step-up in testosterone biosynthesis precursors. Genitography showed blind-ending vagina, and no müllerian derivatives were identified by ultrasonographic studies. Testes are inguinal or intra-abdominal. Because testicular size is dependent on tubular integrity, and therefore is an FSH-dependent function, genetic male patients with Leydig cell hypoplasia have normal or only slightly reduced testicular volume as a result of cryptorchidism. Testicular histology of these patients revealed relatively preserved seminiferous tubules, whereas Leydig cells are not present or appear only as immature forms, indicating a primary defect of Leydig cell development [5, 8].

Milder forms of male sexual abnormalities are also associated with LHCGR mutations that retain some degree of responsiveness to hCG and LH [5, 8–11]. A spectrum of phenotypes was described ranging from incomplete male sexual differentiation characterized by micropenis and/or hypospadias to hypergonadotropic hypogonadism and delayed puberty without ambiguity of the male external genitalia. These patients display elevated levels of serum LH as a result of insufficient negative feedback of gonadal steroid hormones on the anterior pituitary [5].

More recently, unusual inactivating mutations of the *LHCGR* have been reported. A deletion of exon 10 of the *LHCGR* was identified in a patient with normal male phenotype at birth, but no pubertal development [10]. This phenotype suggested that the mutant LHCGR was responsive to fetal hCG, but resistant to pituitary LH. In vitro analysis revealed that the binding affinity for hCG was normal, suggesting that exon 10 is necessary for LH, but not hCG [10, 11].

A novel *LHCGR* gene-inactivating mutation was described involving a cryptic exon located in intron 6 (exon 6A) that caused Leydig cell hypoplasia [2]. The exact role of the cryptic exon 6A is not fully understood. However, when exon 6A is used, it results in truncated LHCGRs consisting of only the first 209 amino acids. Expression of these truncated LHCGRs in heterologous cells leads to intracellular retention of the receptor. To date, two distinct mutations within exon 6A (A557C or G558C) were identified in 46,XY patients with Leydig cell hypoplasia [2].

LH Resistance in Women

Pituitary gonadotropins (LH and FSH) and their receptors are directly involved in the integrated series of events that regulate normal sexual maturation and fertility in women [1, 18]. In the early follicular phase, FSH stimulates follicle growth and induces LH receptor expression on the granulosa cells. Aromatization of androgens under the control of FSH results in progressive estrogen secretion. Subsequently, the mid-cycle LH surge promotes ovulation of the dominant follicle. In the luteal phase, LH induces the formation of the corpus luteum and stimulates progesterone production. Abnormalities in the LHCGR are expected to impair normal folliculogenesis, ovulation and progesterone secretion.

Genetic females with *LHCGR* mutations had female external genitalia, spontaneous scarce to normal pubic hair and normal breast development at puberty. Menarche occurred spontaneously, between 12 and 20 years of age, but usually late, and was followed by menses at variable intervals, ranging from 3 weeks to 15 months, predominantly at intervals of several months [5, 12–14]. One patient with the milder ΔTyr317-Ser324 mutation had normal menses every 28 days from 16 to 20 years, and then developed oligomenorrhea, whereas her sister with the same mutation had oligomenorrhea during all her reproductive life [19]. The patients usually responded to progesterone administration and withdrawal with uterine bleeding [5]. Four patients tried to conceive for at least 1.5 years without success [5, 12, 19].

In 2011, Yariz et al. [20] reported an *LHCGR* mutation identified by whole genome sequencing in two sisters with empty follicle syndrome. This condition has been defined as the failure to retrieve oocytes from mature ovarian follicles after ovulation induction for in vitro fertilization, even after meticulous aspiration and repeated flushing, despite apparently normal follicular development and E_2 levels [21]. These patients had 14–17 years of infertility with apparently normal FSH and estradiol levels and upon stimulation reached estradiol levels above 3,000 pg/ml with several follicles >18 mm, but no oocytes could be retrieved [21, 22]. The only homozygous alteration found by whole exome sequencing that segregated with the empty follicle syndrome phenotype in this family was an *LHCGR* c.1199A>G mutation coding for p.Asn400Ser. Asparagine 400 is highly conserved, and earlier in vitro studies showed that a mutation at this residue results in reduced β-hCG binding to the receptor [21].

Serum LH was high in all patients (10–38 IU/l, normal 0.95–8.4), except in one patient (LH 6.5 mIU/ml) with the milder mutation (ΔTyr317-Ser324), whereas serum FSH was normal or only slightly increased (6.3–11.5 IU/l, normal 2.4–9.3), resulting in a high LH/FSH ratio. Two patients had a gonadotropin-releasing hormone test and responded with high LH peak levels. Estradiol levels ranged from <10 to 122 pg/ml, but were usually lower than 50 pg/ml, levels normally found in the early and mid-follicular phase [23]. One patient underwent an in vitro fertilization attempt, and estradiol levels reached 270 pg/ml with multifollicular development, but no oocyte could be retrieved after hCG stimulation [22]. Progesterone levels ranged from <0.1 to 1.2 ng/ml. Serum prolactin and androgen levels (testosterone, androstenedione, 17-hydroxyprogesterone, DHEA and DHEA-S) were all normal [5, 12–14].

Uterine volume on pelvic ultrasound ranged from small to normal (9–70 ml; normal adult 30–90 ml). Ovarian volume ranged between 3.3 and 22 ml (normal adult 3–9 ml), according to the development of cysts that reached up to 55 mm in diameter. Compared to normal women, these patients had lower estradiol levels despite having larger follicular cysts, indicating reduced steroidogenic efficiency of the follicles. The insufficient estrogen production was corroborated by the high LH levels, indicating inadequate feedback at the hypothalamic-pituitary unit [5, 12–14].

Ovarian biopsy in one patient revealed multiple primordial follicles, preantral follicles with oocytes and few granulosa cell layers, and follicles with a large antrum and well-developed theca cell layer. In these antral follicles, the theca cells had a luteinized appearance, whereas the granulosa cells in the same follicle did not show signs of luteinization. No preovulatory follicles, corpora lutea or corpora albicans were present [13]. Bone density, available in 3 patients, was low in 2 [5, 13] and normal in one patient [12], and was in accordance with estrogen production.

Interestingly, no mutations of the *LHCGR* have been found in a substantial number (30–50%) of patients with the classical phenotype of Leydig cell hypoplasia, or in several women with clinical features of LH resistance, suggesting that genomic defects in other genes may cause gonadotropin resistance and this rare form of abnormal sex development in genetic males [2, 23].

FSH Resistance in Women

Unlike the LH receptor, few natural mutations of the FSHR gene have been described to date. The first inactivating mutation of the FSHR was identified in exon 7 (C566T) in highly inbred Finnish families with autosomal recessive premature ovarian failure and normal karyotype [24]. This mutation was associated with variable pubertal failure and primary or secondary amenorrhea, high serum levels of FSH, and streak or hypoplastic ovaries. Histological examination of the ovaries allowed the detection of follicles. However a block in follicular maturation was observed at early stages. The same natural homozygous mutation of the FSH receptor p.Ala189Val, located in the extracellular domain of the receptor, was found in all affected women. This mutation markedly impaired FSHR function in vitro, consistent with the severe phenotype of the affected patients. The Ala189Val mutation has not been detected in women with a similar phenotype in various countries, suggesting that this mutation is particularly prevalent in the Finnish population because of a founder effect.

More recently, partial phenotype of FSH resistance has also been described. They have secondary amenorrhea with normal puberty, normal-sized ovaries and high serum levels of FSH. Histological and immunocytochemical examination of the ovaries showed a normal follicular development up to the small antral stage and a disruption at further stages. Compound heterozygous of the FSHR were identified which impaired, but did not abolish, receptor in vitro. Interestingly, a correlation between the residual activity of the mutated receptors and the severity of the clinical, biological, and histological phenotypes was observed in these patients.

We investigated the presence of abnormalities in the *FSHR* gene in 15 Brazilian women with familial or sporadic premature ovarian failure [25]. No inactivating mutations were identified in exons 7–10 of these patients. Although the number of Brazilian patients evaluated was small, these findings support the hypothesis that C566T mutation is probably restricted to Finland. We demonstrated a high allelic frequency of two different nucleotide substitutions in exon 10 of the *FSHR* gene, G919A and G2039A, in patients with familial and sporadic premature ovarian failure. These polymorphisms were also found at similar frequencies in normal Brazilian women, indicating these substitutions have no biologic significance.

FSH Resistance in Men

In males, the inactivating mutations of the FSHR receptor have a less clear phenotype. Homozygous males were identified in Finnish families with the Ala189Val mutation [26]. All males were found to be normally masculinized with normal serum testosterone, normal or slightly elevated LH, moderately elevated FSH, and slightly to severely reduced testicular volume. They had abnormal semen parameters ranging from severe or moderate oligozoospermia to normal sperm concentration with a low volume and teratozoospermia. Two men had normal fertility. Conspicuously, none of them was azoospermic. While these findings may potentially suggest that FSH action is not absolutely required for spermatogenesis, it cannot be ruled out that these individuals have some residual FSHR activity. Finally, FSH contributes to testicular size and qualitatively and quantitatively normal spermatogenesis. However, in the presence of normal androgen, fertility is possible in the absence of FSH action.

Conclusions

A spectrum of phenotypes has been associated with inactivating mutations of the LHCG and FSH receptors, closely correlated with the severity of the mutations. The identification and characterization of naturally occurring mutations of the human LH and FSH receptors have considerably advanced our understanding of the actions of these hormones in reproductive physiology, especially in sex differentiation.

Acknowledgments

This work was partially supported by grants from Fundação de Amparo a Pesquisa do Estado de São Paulo – FAPESP No. 05/04726-0 and Conselho Nacional de Desenvolvimento Científico e Tecnológico to I.J.P.A. (300982/2009-7) and A.C.L. (302825/2011-8).

References

1 Ascoli M, Fanelli F, Segaloff DL: The lutropin/choriogonadotropin receptor, a 2002 perspective. Endocr Rev 2002;2:141–174.

2 Kossack N, Simoni M, Richter-Unruh A, Themmen APN, Gromoll J: Mutations in a novel, cryptic exon of the luteinizing hormone/chorionic gonadotropin receptor gene cause male pseudohermaphroditism. PLoS Med 2008;5:e88.

3 Berthezene F, Forest MG, Grimaud JA, Claustrat B, Mornex R: Leydig-cell agenesis: a cause of male pseudohermaphroditism. N Engl J Med 1976;295:969–972.

4 Kremer H, Kraaij R, Toledo SPA, Post M, Fridman JB, Hayashida CY, van Reen M, Milgrom E, Ropers HH, Mariman E, Themmen APN, Brunner HG: Male pseudohermaphroditism due to a homozygous missense mutation of the luteinizing hormone receptor gene. Nat Genet 1995;9:160–164.

5 Latronico AC, Anasti J, Arnhold IJP, Rapaport R, Mendonca BB, Bloise W, Castro M, Tsigos C, Chrousos GP: Testicular and ovarian resistance to luteinizing hormone caused by homozygous inactivating mutations of the luteinizing hormone receptor gene. N Engl J Med 1996;334:507–512.

6 Laue L, Wu SM, Kudo M, Hsueh AJW, Cutler GB Jr, Griffin JE, Wilson JD, Brain C, Berry AC, Grant DB, Chan WY: A nonsense mutation of the human luteinizing hormone receptor gene in Leydig cell hypoplasia. Hum Mol Genet 1995;4:1429–1433.

7 Laue LL, Wu SM, Kudo M, Bourdony CJ, Cutler GB Jr, Hsueh AJW, Chan WY: Compound heterozygous mutations of the luteinizing hormone receptor gene in Leydig cell hypoplasia. Mol Endocrinol 1996;10:987–997.

8 Misrahi M, Meduri G, Pissard S, Bouvattier C, Beau I, Loosfelt H, Jolivet A, Rappaport R, Milgrom E, Bougneres P: Comparison of immunocytochemical and molecular features with the phenotype in a case of incomplete male pseudohermaphroditism associated with a mutation of the luteinizing hormone receptor. J Clin Endocrinol Metab 1997;82:2159–2165.

9 Martens JWM, Verhoef-Post M, Abelin N, Ezabella M, Toledo SPA, Brunner HG, Themmen APN: A homozygous mutation in the luteinizing hormone receptor causes partial Leydig cell hypoplasia: correlation between receptor activity and phenotype. Mol Endocrinol 1998;12:775–783.

10 Gromoll J, Eiholzer U, Nieschlag E, Simoni M: Male hypogonadism caused by homozygous deletion of exon 10 of the luteinizing hormone (LH) receptor: differential action of human chorionic gonadotropin and LH. J Clin Endocrinol Metab 2000;85:2281–2286.

11 Müller T, Gromoll J, Simoni M: Absence of exon 10 of the human luteinizing hormone (LH) receptor impairs LH, but not human chorionic gonadotropin action. J Clin Endocrinol Metab 2003;88:2242–2249.

12 Latronico AC, Chai Y, Arnhold IJP, Liu X, Mendonca BB, Segaloff DL: A homozygous microdeletion in helix seven of the luteinizing hormone receptor associated with familial testicular and ovarian resistance is due to both decreased cell surface expression and impaired Gs activation by the cell surface receptor. Mol Endocrinol 1998;12:442–450.

13 Toledo SPA, Brunner HG, Kraaij R, Post M, Dahia PLM, Hayashida CY, Kremer H, Themmen APN: An inactivating mutation of the luteinizing hormone receptor causes amenorrhea in a 46,XX female. J Clin Endocrinol Metab 1996;81:3850–3854.

14 Stavrou SS, Zhu YS, Cai LQ, Katz MD, Herrera C, Defillo-Ricart M, Imperato-McGinley J: A novel mutation of the human luteinizing hormone receptor in 46XY and 46XX sisters. J Clin Endocrinol Metab 1998;83:2091–2098.

15 Qiao J, Han B, Liu BL, Chen X, Ru Y, Cheng KX, Chen FG, Zhao SX, Liang J, Lu YL, Tang JF, Wu YX, Wu WL, Chen JL, Chen MD, Song HD: A splice site mutation combined with a novel missense mutation of LHCGR cause male pseudohermaphroditism. Hum Mutat 2009;30:E855–E865.

16 Segaloff DL: Diseases associated with mutations of the human lutropin receptor. Prog Mol Biol Transl Sci 2009;89:97–114.

17 Latronico AC, Segaloff DL: Naturally occurring mutations of the luteinizing-hormone receptor: lessons learned about reproductive physiology and G protein-coupled receptors. Am J Hum Genet 1999;65:949–958.

18 Themmen APN: An update of the pathophysiology of human gonadotropin subunit and receptor gene mutations and polymorphisms. Reproduction 2005;130:263–274.

19 Bruysters M, Christin-Maitre S, Verhoef-Post M, Sultan C, Auger J, Faugeron I, Larue L, Lumbroso S, Themmen AP, Bouchard P: A new LH receptor splice mutation responsible for male hypogonadism with subnormal sperm production in the propositus, and infertility with regular cycles in an affected sister. Hum Reprod 2008;23:1917–1923.

20 Yariz KO, Walsh T, Uzak A, Spiliopoulos M, Duman D, Onalan G, King MC, Tekin M: Inherited mutation of the luteinizing hormone/choriogonadotropin receptor (LHCGR) in empty follicle syndrome. Fertil Steril 2011;96:e125–e130.

21 Zreik TG, Garcia-Velasco JA, Vergara TM, Arici A, Olive D, Jones EF: Empty follicle syndrome: evidence for recurrence. Hum Reprod 2000;15: 999–1000.
22 Onalan G, Pabuçcu R, Onalan R, Ceylaner S, Selam B: Empty follicle syndrome in two sisters with three cycles: case report. Hum Reprod 2003;18:1864–1867.
23 Arnhold IJ, Latronico AC, Batista MC, Izzo CR, Mendonca BB: Clinical features of women with resistance to luteinizing hormone. Clin Endocrinol (Oxf) 1999;51:701–707.
24 Aittomäki K, Lucena JL, Pakarinen P, Sistonen P, Tapanainen J, Gromoll J, Kaskikari R, Sankila EM, Lehväslaiho H, Engel AR, Nieschlag E, Huhtaniemi I, de la Chapelle A: Mutation in the follicle-stimulating hormone receptor gene causes hereditary hypergonadotropic ovarian failure. Cell 1995; 82:959–968.
25 da Fonte Kohek MB, Batista MC, Russell AJ, Vass K, Giacaglia LR, Mendonca BB, Latronico AC: No evidence of the inactivating mutation (C566T) in the follicle-stimulating hormone receptor gene in Brazilian women with premature ovarian failure. Fertil Steril 1998;70:565–567.
26 Tapanainen JS, Aittomäki K, Min J, Vaskivuo T, Huhtaniemi IT: Men homozygous for an inactivating mutation of the follicle-stimulating hormone (FSH) receptor gene present variable suppression of spermatogenesis and fertility. Nat Genet 1997;15: 205–206.

Prof. Dr. Ana Claudia Latronico
Laboratório de Hormônios e Genética Molecular LIM/42 Hospital das Clínicas
Disciplina de Endocrinologia Universidade de São Paulo
Av. Dr. Enéas de Carvalho Aguiar, 155, 2° andar, Bloco 6
CEP 05403-900, São Paulo (Brasil)
E-Mail anacl@usp.br

Maghnie M, Loche S, Cappa M, Ghizzoni L, Lorini R (eds): Hormone Resistance and Hypersensitivity. From Genetics to Clinical Management. Endocr Dev. Basel, Karger, 2013, vol 24, pp 33–40 (DOI: 10.1159/000342499)

Clinical and Molecular Aspects of Androgen Insensitivity

Olaf Hiort

Division of Experimental Pediatric Endocrinology and Diabetes, Department of Pediatrics and Adolescent Medicine, Universität zu Lübeck, Lübeck, Germany

Abstract

Androgen insensitivity describes the inability of cells to respond adequately to androgens. The clinical aspects are well characterized and described in the androgen insensitivity syndrome, where underandrogenization occurs despite normal to high levels of androgens. In 46,XY individuals, this is associated with a variable phenotype ranging from completely female to ambiguous genitalia and infertility in males with gynecomastia. Androgen action is facilitated by a single androgen receptor (AR), whose gene is localized on the X chromosome. However, the identification of mutations in the AR gene in patients with androgen insensitivity is variable, and chances are lower the more subtle the phenotype is. Therefore, other currently unknown mechanisms must be hypothesized to lead to the respective phenotype. The AR is a nuclear transcription factor, acting in concert with an array of only partly known cofactors serving as modulators of target gene transcription. The induced transcription pattern is highly tissue and cell specific, and in some tissues may lead to lasting changes of cell programming. Only one regulated gene APOD has currently been identified to serve as a clinical tool for the diagnosis of androgen insensitivity.

Amongst the 'disorders of sex development' (DSD), androgen insensitivity syndromes (AIS) are a common cause of underandrogenization in 46,XY individuals [1]. They are diagnosed clinically, because at the time of assessment, apparently the capability of the testes to synthesize adequate amounts of testosterone is perceived as within the male reference interval for age; however, the responsiveness to these androgens is diminished [2]. The unresponsiveness to androgens can be quite variable; therefore, the range of phenotype is broad. Three categories have been crudely described in 46,XY children: a complete AIS with a completely female appearance of the external genitalia, a partial AIS with a variable degree of genital ambiguity ranging from hypospadias in a child reared male to a slight virilization in a child reared female, and a minimal AIS in children with isolated micropenis without any urethral abnormality. At the time of puberty, the phenotype is more distinct, as patients with complete AIS may sometimes develop some degree of sexual hair, while in others the secondary sexual hair is completely absent. In partial AIS, at puberty a degree of virilization in combination with feminization is seen; also the patients assigned male mostly develop striking gynecomastia. Minimal AIS is also usually associated with gynecomastia as well as a variable degree of spermatogenic failure. Therefore, Quigley et al. [2] and Sinnecker et al. [3] describe up to 7 different clinical categories in AIS. This knowledge is important for the understanding of AIS, especially for counseling of affected individuals. The management of AIS includes: adequate disclosure; assessment of the need of hormone therapy, especially in males with partial and minimal AIS as well as in females whose gonads have been removed; evaluation of the possibility of benign and malignant tumors of the gonads; the need for genital operations, and of utmost importance, the psychological counseling of the affected and their families.

Androgen-Dependent Genital Development

The sex-specific development of the embryo and fetus is initially controlled by the genetic steps leading to the differentiation of the bipotent gonad into either testis or ovary. Subsequently, sexual differentiation mainly depends on hormonal influences [for review see 4]. While anti-Müller hormone, secreted from Sertoli cells, leads to regression of the müllerian ducts, testosterone, normally secreted from the testicular Leydig cells stabilizes the wolffian ducts with differentiation of epididymis, vasa deferentia, and seminal vesicles. The external differentiation of male genitalia requires the conversion of testosterone to dihydrotestosterone (DHT). DHT will induce closure of the urethral groves and outgrowth onto the tip of the phallus, fusion of the labioscrotal folds, as well as provoke the growth of the phallus during fetal life. Thus, androgen synthesis is high during the prenatal period in order to induce the spatial and time-dependent genital development. The influence of androgen levels on genital differentiation is demonstrated clinically by the appearance of 46,XX patients with hyperandrogenization such as in congenital adrenal hyperplasia, as well as in 46,XY patients with androgen biosynthesis defects leading to underandrogenization. AIS is peculiar in that testicular function is apparently normal leading to regression of Müller structures and apparently adequate levels of testosterone. Thus, it is a disorder which affects the peripheral target cell with its machinery to respond adequately to androgens. Today, only one single androgen receptor (AR) has been identified in humans. This AR acts as a nuclear transcription factor and is expressed from the 8th week of gestation, thus controlling the sexual differentiation in response to the rising androgen levels.

Genetics and Molecular Biology

As the major members of the group of nuclear receptors, the AR is composed of three major functional domains, namely the ligand-binding domain (LBD), the DNA-binding domain (DBD), as well as a large N-terminal end, which serves as a regulating element, with a hinge region between the LBD and the DBD [2]. The AR exerts its action with binding of the ligand in the cytoplasm, where it is bound to heat shock proteins and cochaperones [4]. The AR then undergoes conformational changes with the parts of the LBD forming the activation function 2 (AF2). An activation function 1 exists in the N-terminal domain, which is ligand independent. The AF2 links with the N-terminal transactivation domain in an intramolecular interaction through the utilization of an ^{23}FQNLF^{27} motif at binding of the hormone, whereby the heat shock proteins are dissociated and the receptor translocates to the nucleus. The AR then joins a second AR hormone complex to form a homodimer and binds to specific androgen response elements in defined target genes [4]. It controls the transcription machinery in concert with a lot of coregulators, which may be very cell specific; thus, the individual cellular response is highly target and maybe also time specific in regulating the transcriptional expression of the target genes [5]. Also, different androgens have different binding capabilities, and may lead to a different cellular reaction [6]. Therefore, this single AR can elicit an array of many differentially regulated responses. The crystal structure of the DBD and LBD of the AR has been elucidated, and it is composed of 12 α-helices and 4 β-helices, which form an α-helical sandwich, a structure seen also in other steroid hormone receptors.

The AR gene is located on the X-chromosome at Xq11–12, and it is encoded by 8 exons, where a first large exon is translated into the N-terminal domain, while exons 2 and 3 encode for the DBD and exons 4–8 for the LBD [2]. The whole gene has a length of approximately 90 kb; however, the transcribed region is only about 2,750 bp in length, coding for a protein with a variable length of about 920 amino acids, corresponding to a molecular weight of 110–112 kDa. The variability of the coding region is the result of two polymorphic trinucleotid repeat regions, which are localized in the first exons, namely a CAG and a GGN repeat. The role of the trinucleotid repeats has been discussed extensively both with respect to the cellular functions of the AR as well as their potential role in human disorders [7]. In general, longer CAG repeats have been found to diminish transactivation capacity of the receptor, while shorter CAG repeat length may lead to enhanced transactivation. Hyperexpansion of the CAG or polyglutamine stretch to more than 38 residues is associated with a specific neuromuscular disorder termed spinobulbar muscular atrophy or Kennedy diseases [2]. Affected patients were found to have signs of minimal AIS with gynecomastia and impaired fertility. Furthermore, the length of the polymorphic repeats may have an influence also on the transactivation potential of any mutated receptor in partial androgen insensitivity [7].

Genetics in Androgen Insensitivity Syndromes

With the identification and characterization of the AR gene, mutations within the coding region have been identified associated with all forms of AIS. More than 800 different mutations have been recorded in the international AR gene mutation database (www.mcgill/androgendb/), with most of them point mutations leading to amino acid substitutions in the protein structure. However, splice site mutations, and also complete deletions, as well as small insertion and deletions, and substitution mutations leading to premature termination of the protein are reported. While the latter are nearly always associated with complete AIS, the amino acid substitutions can be associated with complete, partial or minimal AIS, depending on the site of the mutation and the residue exchanged [4, 7–9]. Due to the hemizygous inheritance pattern, de novo mutations are as frequent as in autosomal-dominant disorders and may comprise up to 30% of the cases [10]. This is of importance for genetic counseling, but in the case of somatic de novo mutations may also affect the phenotype of the patient and, hence, influences therapeutic decision-making.

For many mutations, the deleterious effects have been proved through detailed in vitro studies. For novel mutations, this should be performed by recreating the mutation in an appropriate expression vector and study of the impact on transactivation employing cotransfection of an androgen-responsive reporter gene in an AR-negative mammalian cell line. Usually, the analysis includes hormone binding of the mutant, as well as protein stability, nuclear transport, and in some cases DNA binding [8]. Also, the effects of different androgens and different promoters of the AR responsive genes can give novel insights into the pathogenicity of any mutant. At this time, however, these studies do not explain the highly variable phenotypes seen with the same mutation in many reported cases of partial AIS. Mutations leading to these phenotypes often affect ligand binding, but also chaperone interactions, and may alter posttranslational modifications of the receptor. With a partial residual function of the mutant, cell-dependent expression of coactivators and corepressors of the AR is particular important and might be modulated very differently. Therefore, in the case of these mutants, the use of different reporter genes and cell lines may be necessary to investigate the pathogenicity of such a variation [8].

While the mammalian cell-based in vitro assays give some insight into the molecular pathology of a given mutation of the AR, for individualized purposes the characterization of target gene profiles in cells derived from patients with AIS is of high interest [11]. The use of genome-wide analysis of genital skin fibroblasts from patients with proved AR mutations has identified distinct androgen-regulated gene profiles which are independent of the chromosomal sex, but correlate with the genital phenotype of these patients [12]. Also in peripheral blood monocytes, a tissue initially thought to be sex independent, specific androgen-dependent expression patterns could be assessed [13]. The expression patterns found were independent of the current status of hormone therapy; therefore, it can be concluded that androgenization during sexual development of the embryo leads to a specific androgen-related 'fingerprint' in the expression pattern of both genital and non-genital target tissues. This pattern will persist during the life of this individual and cannot be altered again. This view is particularly important also in clinical decision-making, because it implies that any postnatal intervention cannot change but only partly modulate the androgen phenotype in the patient. For diagnostic purposes, the identification of Apolipoprotein D as a highly specific androgen-regulated gene in genital skin mesenchymal cells in response to DHT treatment is promising, as this marker may be used specifically for the diagnosis of AIS even in the absence of the detection of a relevant mutation in the AR and differentiate this form of DSD from others [14].

Clinical Management

In infants and children, the initial diagnosis of AIS is difficult. Laboratory values are mostly inconclusive, and usually show a 'normal' testicular function according to age-related reference intervals. In patients with complete AIS, there may be even low values for LH and testosterone during the so-called mini-puberty, and only after LHRH stimulation is there a strong rise in gonadotropins and also in testosterone [15, 16]. In some cases of partial AIS, testosterone levels may even be elevated. During puberty, the diagnosis often becomes clearer because normal to elevated LH levels are found in conjunction with rising and even above the male reference interval lying testosterone levels despite a lack of androgenization as seen in the clinical investigation of the patient [17]. So, after puberty, AIS is a clinical diagnosis depending on the typical phenotype with underandrogenization and feminization. Only after structured clinical assessment and appropriate laboratory and imaging investigations (including laparoscopy) should detailed molecular genetic studies be ordered.

The diagnosis of a DSD is often seen as very disturbing for a patient and the family [18]. It has been agreed upon that the disclosure of any DSD diagnosis, as well as the discussion of the diagnostic steps and the counseling of further management requires an expert multidisciplinary team, consisting of a pediatric endocrinologist, a pediatric surgeon or urologist, a psychologist, a geneticist and several other subspecialties, depending on the need for this individual [1]. These include specialists in gonadal pathology, laboratory medicine, gynecology or neonatology, depending on the age of the patient, urology and internal medicine. The multidisciplinary team may be completed with an ethicist and a socioreligious counsel for the family, as patients and their families may come from different cultural backgrounds.

The German Ethical Council of the German Parliament recently published recommendations for dealing with patients with DSD, and favored the implementation of competence centers, which act as tertiary care centers for both patients and also physicians requiring additional help (www.ethikrat.org/intersexualitaet). The competence centers are then urged to act professionally in defining structured diagnostic pathways, but also to inform both patients and caring physicians about their management possibilities in full disclosure. Furthermore, the centers are the hubs for linking appropriate research with clinical care and should provide structured teaching to health care professionals, namely physicians, nurses and midwifes, who may be confronted in dealing with DSD patients and their families.

With respect to AIS, current management strategies opt for as little interventions as possible with as much as absolutely necessary. In the cases of partial AIS with female sex assignment, this should include the options for genital surgery. The current statements point towards deferring genital operations to a time when the patient can give informed consent and the gender identity is stable. Therefore, in contrast to current management in congenital adrenal hyperplasia, genital surgery in partial AIS females may be performed late. Controversial is the management of patients with partial AIS, who have been assigned to a male sex. As in other cases of hypospadias, the repair is usually favored in the first year of life. In complete AIS, often genital surgery is not necessary. Some patients may require elongation of the vagina, but this should be decided on the basis of informed consent after the patient has reached adulthood and wants to be sexually active.

In recent years, dramatic changes have occurred regarding the management of the gonads in AIS. In patients with a female or almost female phenotype, corresponding to complete AIS or partial AIS, the gonads are left in situ until the patient can give consent to the management procedures. In cases with partial AIS and female sex assignment at birth, decision-making should be discussed at the onset of puberty. In the case of a stable female gender identity of the patient, gonads may still be removed to prevent unwanted virilization. If there is still uncertainty about gender in the patient, puberty may be postponed with the use of GnRH analogues.

In patients with complete AIS, the gonads should be left in situ throughout puberty and maybe also beyond. The overall prevalence of testicular malignancies may be below 1% [19]. However, as there are no regular registries available to record the development of benign or malignant tumors, a structured regular assessment of the gonads should be offered, e.g. with regular ultrasound every 6 months with the start of puberty.

If the gonads are removed in patients with complete AIS, usually a monotherapy with continuous estrogens is used for hormone replacement to maintain secondary sexual characteristics and to promote physical and social well-being [20]. However, this has been challenged by some patients with complete AIS, who reported that this would not correspond to their typical hormone profiles and that they felt diminished in their health-related quality of life [21]. Some women with complete AIS have started with a high-dose testosterone therapy, but this practice remains anecdotal until a recently started double-blind clinical trial employing testosterone versus estradiol therapy in complete AIS has been evaluated (www.cais-studie.de). The management of hormone therapy in partial AIS and other forms of DSD may also change in the near future depending on the outcome of this trial.

To gain better understanding and knowledge of the diagnosis of all forms of DSD including AIS, international collaborations have been established including both clinical and research-based networks. This collaboration includes an international DSD database which allows the anonymized registration of all cases of DSD with clinical descriptions and possible diagnosis to allow the exchange of data and biomaterials between centers according to the specified consent of the patients [22]. This database termed I-DSD arose from a recent European collaborative study funded by the 7th EU Framework Programme, and should provide the basis for successful future research and hopefully also for respective clinical trials.

Acknowledgment

The author has received funding from the European Community's Seventh Framework Programme under Grant Agreement No. 201444 (EuroDSD) as well as from the German Ministry of Education and Research (BMBF 01KG1003).

References

1 Hughes IA, Houk C, Ahmed SF, Lee PA, LWPES Consensus Group, ESPE Consensus Group: Consensus statement on management of intersex disorders. Arch Dis Child 2006;91:554–563.

2 Quigley CA, De Bellis A, Marschke KB, El-Awady M, Wilson EM, French FS: Androgen receptor defects: historical, clinical and molecular perspectives. Endocr Rev 1995;16:271–322.

3 Sinnecker GH, Hiort O, Nitsche EM, Holterhus PM, Kruse K: Functional assessment and clinical classification of androgen sensitivity in patients with mutations of the androgen receptor gene. German Collaborative Intersex Study Group. Eur J Pediatr 1997;156:7–14.

4 Werner R, Grötsch H, Hiort O: 46,XY disorders of sex development – the undermasculinised male with disorders of androgen action. Best Pract Res Clin Endocrinol Metab 2010;24:263–277.

5 Grötsch H, Kunert M, Mooslehner KA, Gao Z, Struve D, Hughes IA, Hiort O, Werner R: RWDD1 interacts with the ligand binding domain of the androgen receptor and acts as a coactivator of androgen-dependent transactivation. Mol Cell Endocrinol 2012;358:53–62.

6 Holterhus PM, Piefke S, Hiort O: Anabolic steroids, testosterone-precursors and virilizing androgens induce distinct activation profiles of androgen responsive promoter constructs. J Steroid Biochem Molec Biol 2002;82:269–275.

7 Werner R, Holterhus PM, Binder G, Schwarz HP, Morlot M, Struve D, Marschke C, Hiort O: The A645D mutation in the hinge region of the human AR gene modulates AR activity depending on the context of the polymorphic glutamine and glycine repeats. J Clin Endocrinol Metab 2006;91:3515–3520.

8 Werner R, Zhan J, Gesing J, Struve D, Hiort O: In-vitro characterization of androgen receptor mutations associated with complete androgen insensitivity syndrome reveals distinct functional deficits. Sex Dev 2008;2:73–83.

9 Hiort O, Holterhus PM, Horter T, Schulze W, Kremke B, Bals-Pratsch M, Sinnecker GHG, Kruse K: Significance of mutations in the androgen receptor gene in males with idiopathic infertility. J Clin Endocrinol Metab 2000;85:2810–2815.

10 Hiort O, Sinnecker GHG, Holterhus PM, Nitsche EM, Kruse K: Inherited and de novo androgen receptor gene mutations: investigation of single-case families. J Pediatr 1998;131:939–943.

11 Holterhus PM, Hiort O, Demeter J, Brown PO, Brooks JD: Differential gene expression patterns in genital fibroblasts of normal and 46,XY-females with androgen insensitivity syndrome: evidence for early programming involving the androgen receptor. Genome Biol 2003;4:R37.

12 Holterhus PM, Deppe U, Werner R, Richter-Unruh A, Bebermeier JH, Wunsch L, Krege S, Schweikert HU, Demeter J, Riepe F, Hiort O, Brooks JD: Intrinsic androgen-dependent gene expression patterns revealed by comparison of genital fibroblasts from normal males and individuals with complete and partial androgen insensitivity syndrome. BMC Genomics 2007;18:376.

13 Holterhus PM, Bebermeier JH, Werner R, Demeter J, Richter-Unruh A, Cario G, Appari M, Siebert R, Riepe F, Brooks JD, Hiort O: Disorders of sex development expose transcriptional autonomy of genetic sex and androgen-programmed hormonal sex in human blood leukocytes. BMC Genomics 2009; 10:292.

14 Appari M, Werner R, Wünsch L, Cario G, Demeter J, Hiort O, Riepe F, Brooks JD, Holterhus PM: Apolipoprotein D (APOD) is a putative biomarker of androgen receptor function in androgen insensitivity syndrome. J Mol Med 2009;87:623–632.

15 Bouvattier C, Carel JC, Lecointre C, David A, Sultan C, Bertrand AM, Morel Y, Chaussain JL: Postnatal changes of T, LH, and FSH in 46,XY infants with mutations in the AR gene. J Clin Endocrinol Metab 2002;87:29–32.

16 Ahmed SF, Cheng A, Hughes IA: Assessment of the gonadotrophin-gonadal axis in androgen insensitivity syndrome. Arch Dis Child 1999;80:324–329.

17 Papadimitriou DT, Linglart A, Morel Y, Chaussain JL: Puberty in subjects with complete androgen insensitivity syndrome. Horm Res 2006;65:126–131.

18 Köhler B, Kleinemeier E, Lux A, Hiort O, Grüters A, Thyen U, the DSD Network Working Group: Satisfaction with genital surgery and sexual life of adults with XY disorders of sex development: results from the German Clinical Evaluation Study. J Clin Endocrinol Metab 2012;97:577–588.

19 Cools M, Wolffenbuttel KP, Drop SL, Oosterhuis JW, Looijenga LH: Gonadal development and tumor formation at the crossroads of male and female sex determination. Sex Dev 2011;5:167–180.

20 Warne GL, Grover S, Zajac JD: Hormonal therapies for individuals with intersex conditions: protocol for use. Treat Endocrinol 2005;4:19–29.

21 Bertelloni S, Dati E, Baroncelli GI, Hiort O: Hormonal management of complete androgen insensitivity syndrome from adolescence onward. Horm Res Paediatr 2011;76:428–433.

22 Ahmed SF, Rodie M, Jiang J, Sinnott RO: The European disorder of sex development registry: a virtual research environment. Sex Dev 2010;4:192–198.

Prof. Dr. Olaf Hiort
Division of Pediatric Endocrinology and Diabetes
Department of Pediatrics, University of Lübeck
Ratzeburger Allee 160, DE–23538 Lübeck (Germany)
E-Mail hiort@paedia.ukl.mu-luebeck.de

Maghnie M, Loche S, Cappa M, Ghizzoni L, Lorini R (eds): Hormone Resistance and Hypersensitivity. From Genetics to Clinical Management. Endocr Dev. Basel, Karger, 2013, vol 24, pp 41–56 (DOI: 10.1159/000342502)

Exploring the Molecular Mechanisms of Glucocorticoid Receptor Action from Sensitivity to Resistance

Sivapriya Ramamoorthy · John A. Cidlowski

Laboratory of Signal Transduction, National Institute of Environmental Health Sciences, National Institutes of Health, Department of Health and Human Services, Research Triangle Park, N.C., USA

Abstract

Glucocorticoids regulate a variety of physiological processes, and are commonly used to treat disorders of inflammation, autoimmune diseases, and cancer. Glucocorticoid action is predominantly mediated through the classic glucocorticoid receptor (GR), but sensitivity to glucocorticoids varies among individuals, and even within different tissues from the same individual. The molecular basis of this phenomenon can be partially explained through understanding the process of generating bioavailable ligand and the molecular heterogeneity of the GR. The molecular mechanisms that regulate glucocorticoid action highlight the dynamic nature of hormone signaling and provide novel insights into genomic glucocorticoid actions and glucocorticoid sensitivity. Although glucocorticoids are highly effective for therapeutic purposes, long-term and/or high-dose glucocorticoid administration often leads to reduced glucocorticoid sensitivity or resistance. Here, we summarize our current understanding of the mechanisms that modulate glucocorticoid sensitivity and resistance with a focus on GR-mediated signaling.

Glucocorticoids are a class of stress-induced steroid hormones synthesized by the adrenal cortex under control of the hypothalamic-pituitary-adrenal axis [1]. Endogenous glucocorticoid levels in the serum display a classic circadian pattern, peaking at the beginning of the period of highest activity. Additionally, glucocorticoid levels are strongly elevated in response to a variety of physical and psychological stresses [1]. Cortisol in humans and corticosterone in rodents act to regulate diverse cellular functions including development, homeostasis, metabolism, cognition and inflammation. Glucocorticoids play a significant role in maintaining the immune system, acting to prevent excessive and harmful responses to injury or infection. The anti-inflammatory and immunomodulatory properties underlie the use of glucocorticoids in the clinic where they are used to treat inflammatory diseases and oncological disorders [1].

A plethora of synthetic glucocorticoids have been developed for therapeutic use, and the worldwide market in oral and topical glucocorticoids is estimated to be worth more than USD 10 billion per year [2]. Glucocorticoid agonists are frequently used to treat many inflammatory conditions, from inflammatory arthritis, ulcerative colitis to asthma and skin diseases. Proapoptotic properties of glucocorticoids make them a major component of chemotherapeutic regimens for the treatment of cancers of hematological origins including Hodgkin's lymphoma, acute lymphoblastic leukemia (ALL) and multiple myelomas. Glucocorticoid usage continues to grow every year, driven by increased prevalence of chronic diseases in an ageing population and by increased duration of treatment in certain patients. Although glucocorticoids are highly effective for therapeutic purposes, long-term and/or high-dose glucocorticoid administration is commonly associated with adverse side effects, like hyperglycemia, weight gain, hypertension, osteoporosis, depression and decreased immunological function. Furthermore, patients on glucocorticoids can develop reduced glucocorticoid sensitivity and even resistance. Current research is focused on developing synthetic glucocorticoids with increased tissue selectivity to minimize the side effects by dissociating the desired anti-inflammatory effects from undesirable side effects [3]. Here, we summarize the recent advances and molecular processes involved in glucocorticoid sensitivity and function and discuss in detail the mechanisms that contribute to glucocorticoid resistance. The potential role of glucocorticoid receptor (GR) gene in determining cellular responsiveness to glucocorticoids is emphasized.

The Glucocorticoid Receptor

Organization of the hGR Gene, mRNA and Protein

Glucocorticoids mediate their effect through intracellular GR, which belongs to a large family of transcription factors known as the nuclear hormone receptors. The human GR (NR3C1) is the product of one gene that is located in chromosome 5q31–32. The hGR promoter lacks a consensus TATA box and CCAAT motif, however contains binding sites for transcription factors like AP1, SP1, AP2 nuclear factor-κB (NF-κB) and CREB. The hGR gene consists of 9 exons; exon 1 forms the 5′-untranslated region, while exon 2–9 code for the GR protein. Recent studies have identified 9 alternative first exons (1A, 1B, 1C, 1D, 1E, 1F, 1H, 1I, and 1J) that are generated from unique promoter usage, and likely account for tissue-specific expression of GR. Exon 2 forms the N-terminal domain of GR, exon 3–4 form the central DNA-binding domain (DBD), while exons 5–9 code for the ligand-binding domain (LBD; fig. 1a).

Alternative splicing of the hGR gene in exon 9 generates two highly homologous mRNA transcripts that results in the production of two GR isoforms termed GRα and GRβ. Both the isoforms contain exons 1–8 with different version of exon 9, exon 9α and -β, respectively. The two isoforms are identical up to amino acid 727, but vary beyond this position. The predominant form of GR (GRα) is a protein composed of 777 amino acids. In GRβ, the carboxy terminal 50 amino acids of GRα are replaced by 15 non-homologous amino acids [4].

Our laboratory has identified N-terminal isoforms of GR, which are generated by alternative translation initiation. In 2001, Yudt and Cidlowski [5] demonstrated that COS-1 cells transiently transfected with cDNA encoding hGRα, yield two GR proteins of 94 and 91 kDa termed hGR-A and hGR-B, respectively. Subsequent analysis revealed that hGRα mRNA is translated from at least eight alternative initiation sites producing multiple GRα isoforms termed GR-A, B, C1, C2, C3, D1, D2 and D3. The 94-kDa protein is the classic GRα which is now termed GRα-A, the 91-kDa protein is GRα-B, the 82- to 84-kDa proteins form GRα-C1, C2 and C3, and the 53- to 56-kDa proteins produce D1, D2 and D3 (fig. 1a). The internal AUG codons for all the isoforms are conserved among the human, rat and mouse gene. The mechanism for generating the translational isoforms involves leaky 5′ ribosomal scanning and/or ribosomal shunting, both of which are regulated by mRNA-specific elements. Since all the alternative start codons are located in the amino terminal half of the receptor, hGR-α isoforms have identical DBD and LBD, but differ at their N-terminal region [6].

Similar to other steroid hormone receptors, GR is a modular protein organized into three major functional domains: the N-terminal domain, the central DBD and the C-terminal LBD. The N-terminal domain covering amino acids 1–420 is poorly conserved and is the most variable domain between the steroid hormone receptors. The N-terminal domain contains the transactivation domain AF-1 (activation function-1), which activates target genes in a ligand-independent fashion. The central domain is highly conserved and harbors the DBD, which contains two zinc finger motifs. The carboxy-terminal of GR contains the LBD (aa 527–777), which recognizes and binds ligand. A second activation function domain AF-2 is located within this carboxy-terminal region. The C-terminus also contains sequences important for interaction with heat shock proteins and coregulators (fig. 1b).

The classic mode of action of steroids occurs by direct regulation of gene transcription. In the absence of ligand, GRα is mainly found in the cytoplasm as a heterocomplex by coordinated associations with molecular chaperones, such as heat shock proteins 40 (hsp40), hsp70 and hsp90, and cochaperones including hsp70-interacting protein (hip) and hsp70/hsp90-organizing protein (hop). These chaperones maintain the receptor in the proper confirmation to bind the ligand in a hydrophobic pocket in the C-terminus. When lipophilic glucocorticoids diffuse across the plasma membrane and bind GR, this induces

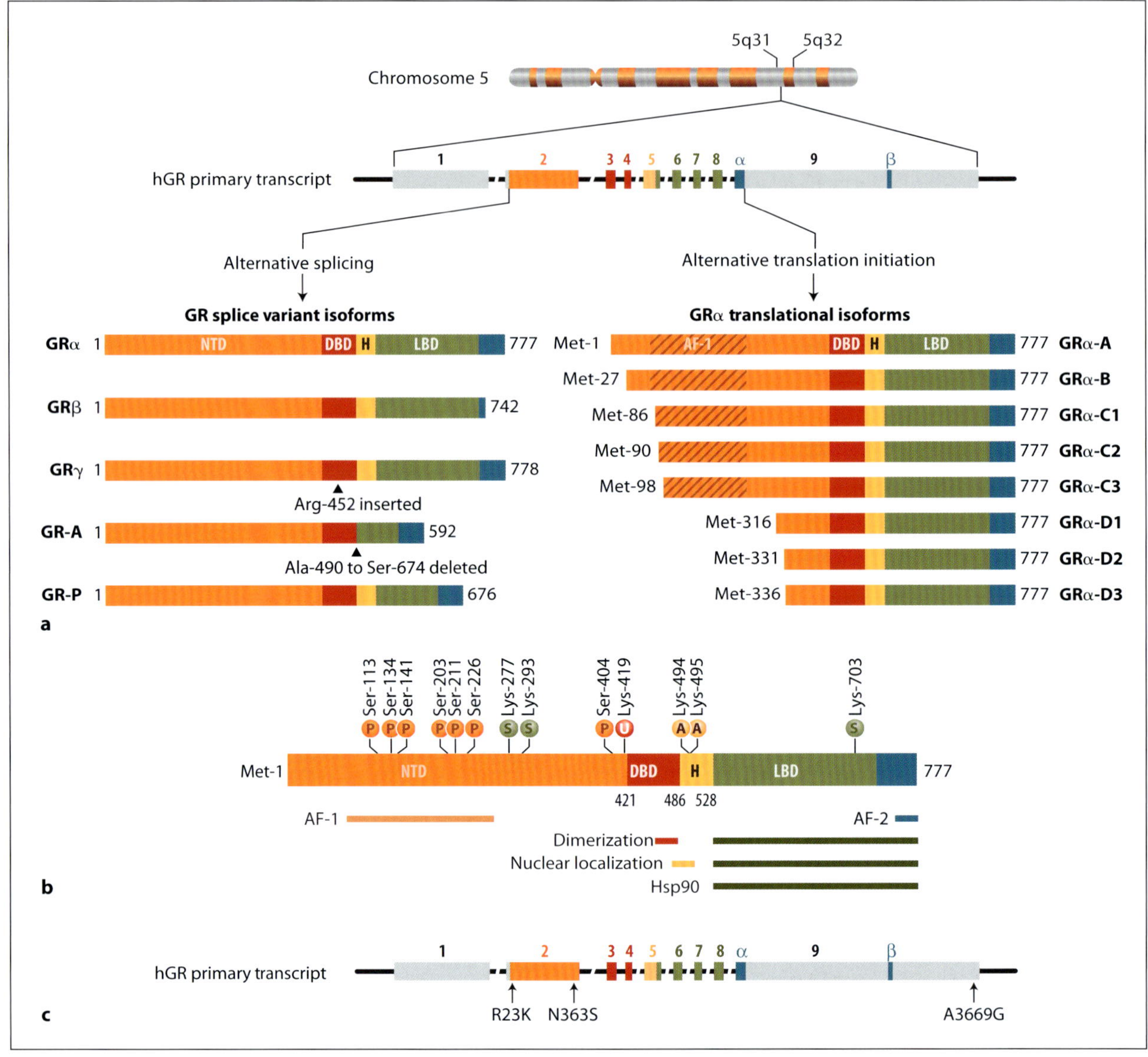

Fig. 1. Genomic location and organization of the human GR. **a** Alternative splicing and translation initiation of hGR primary transcript. The hGR gene (NR3C1) is one locus on chromosome 5q31–32. The hGR primary transcript is composed of 9 exons, with exon 2 encoding most of the N-terminal domain (NTD), exons 3 and 4 encoding the DBD, and exons 5–9 encoding the hinge region (H) and LBD. GR splice variant isoform: The classic GRα protein results from splicing of exon 8 to the beginning of exon 9. GRβ is produced from an alternative splice acceptor site that links the end of exon 8 to downstream sequences in exon 9, encoding a variant with a unique 15 amino acid at C terminus (positions 728–742). GRγ is generated by an alternative splice donor site in the intronic sequence separating exons 3 and 4, resulting in a protein with an arginine insertion (Arg-452) between the two zinc fingers of the DBD. GR-A is produced from alternative splicing that joins exon 4 to exon 8, deleting the proximal 185 amino acids of the LBD (Ala-490-Ser-674) encoded by exons 5–7. GR-P is formed by a failure to splice exon 7 to exon 8. The retained intronic sequence introduces a stop codon, resulting in a truncated receptor mutant missing the distal half of the LBD. GRα translational iso-

rearrangement of the GR heterocomplex leading to GR homodimerization and nuclear translocation. Once inside the nucleus, GR can regulate transcription positively or negatively [7].

Transcriptional Activation by the Glucocorticoid Receptor

Once inside the nucleus, GR binds directly to DNA elements called glucocorticoid response elements (GREs) to stimulate target gene expression. Binding to GRE induces conformational changes in GR leading to coordinated recruitment of coactivators and chromatin-remodeling complexes that influence the activity of RNA polymerase II and activate gene transcription (fig. 2). The classic view that GR induces gene expression by binding to GREs located only in the promoter proximal region of the target gene has been questioned by recent discoveries using ChIP-chip and next-generation sequencing (ChIP-seq) [8]. In these studies, GR-binding sites are isolated by chromatin immunoprecipitation and then identified by ChIP-seq or by hybridization to tile microarray. The comprehensive genomic map of GR:DNA binding derived from these studies revealed that many GR-binding sites identified are located far from the promoter proximal region of target genes and showed an unexpected difference between the activation and repressive functions of the GR. A significant proportion of the GR-binding sites lacked a consensus GRE element, which suggests that binding of GR to the chromatin may in many cases occur by tethering to other transcription factors [8]. Additionally, GR can physically interact with the members of the signal transducer and activator of transcription (STAT) family, either in conjunction with binding a GRE or apart, to enhance transcription of certain target genes. What remains to be established, however, is the functionality of these distant GR-binding sites in relation to the transcription of genes or other undiscovered functions encoded in the GR protein.

In contrast to the classic model where binding of transcription factors to DNA is characterized by stable complexes, the binding of GR to chromatin and the hormone-dependent remodeling of chromatin are highly dynamic and differentially affected by

forms: Domain organization of the GRα translational isoforms. Initiation of translation from eight different AUG start codons in a single GR-mRNA generates receptor isoforms with progressively shorter N-terminal domains. This generates the GRα translational isoforms GRα-A, B, C1, C2, C3, D1, D2 and D3. **b** Domain structure and posttranslational modifications of hGR-α. GR contains three major functional regions, the N-terminal transactivation domain (NTD), the central DBD and the C-terminal LBD. The region located between the DBD and LBD is known as the hinge region (H). Regions involved in transcriptional activation (AF1 and AF2), dimerization, nuclear localization and chaperone hsp90 binding are indicated. Sites of posttranslational modifications like phosphorylation (P), sumoylation (S), ubiquitination (U) and acetylation (A) are indicated. **c** hGR polymorphisms. Arrows indicate polymorphisms that result in amino acid changes and A3669G which leads to GR stability.

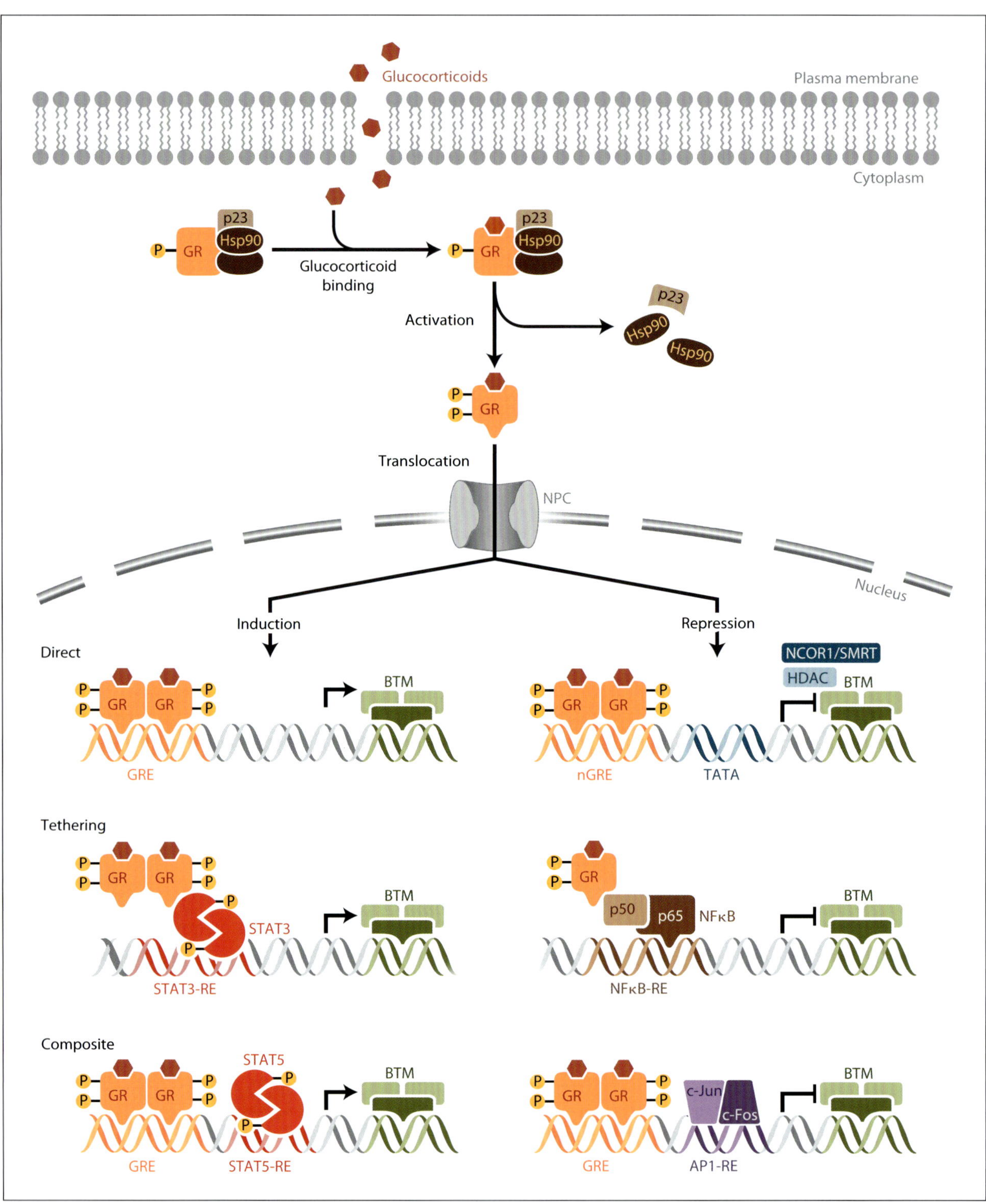
Glucocorticoids
Plasma membrane
Cytoplasm
p23
Hsp90
GR
P
Glucocorticoid binding
Activation
Hsp90
Translocation
NPC
Nucleus
Induction
Repression
Direct
BTM
GRE
NCOR1/SMRT
HDAC
nGRE
TATA
Tethering
STAT3
STAT3-RE
p50
p65
NFκB
NFκB-RE
Composite
STAT5
STAT5-RE
c-Jun
c-Fos
AP1-RE

ligand type. Using fluorescently tagged receptor coupled with photo-bleaching experiments, GR was found to rapidly cycle on and off the chromatin in living cells within seconds to minutes. Even though various important findings have emerged from these large-scale GR-chromatin interaction studies, several questions still remain to be addressed. GR-chromatin binding data alone do not prove that the binding of GR at a specific site is important in the regulation of a particular target gene. Therefore, a combination of location analysis and expression profiling is required to validate if GR binding sites are functional.

Glucocorticoid-induced gene expression is frequently cell type-specific and only a small proportion of genes are commonly activated between different tissues. Tissue-specific target gene activation by glucocorticoids has been shown to be dependent on accessibility of the GR-binding site which in turn is determined by DNA methylation and higher order chromatin structures like long-range chromatin loops. Thus, tissue-specific target gene activation may be determined by the tissue-specific chromatin landscape, which influences binding of GR to the cognate DNA elements.

Transcriptional regulation of GR is also modulated by recruitment of coactivators, which mediate posttranslation modifications of histones (acetylation and methylation). This property aids in altering the chromatin structure and recruiting other cofactors, thus making the chromatin more accessible for the assembly of general transcription factors and the RNA polymerase complex at the target gene promoter. The identity of coregulators that contribute to GR transactivation has grown in the recent years to numbers in the hundreds. Some of the well-studied GR coactivators are the SRC family proteins, mediator complex and SWI/SNF complexes [7]. It has been shown that binding of liganded GR to the GRE results in a conformational change that facilitates the binding of SRC to GR and cooperates in the assembly of the transcription initiation complex at the promoter of the target gene.

Posttranslational modifications of GR further modulate the transcriptional landscape of the receptor. Phosphorylation is the most studied covalent modification of GR. At least seven serine residues (Ser-113, Ser-134, Ser-141, Ser-203, Ser-211, Ser-226 and Ser-404) are phosphorylated in GR, and all these sites are also conserved in mouse and rat (fig. 1b). Other sites of phosphorylation include Ser-45 and 267 [9]. The receptor displays a basal level of phosphorylation and becomes hyperphosphorylated upon binding glucocorticoids. Phosphorylation of GRα changes its transcriptional activity, often in a gene-specific manner. Ligand-dependent phosphorylation

Fig. 2. Genomic action of GR. Upon binding glucocorticoids, cytoplasmic GR undergoes a conformation change (activation), becomes hyper-phosphorylated (P), dissociates from heterocomplex, and translocates into the nucleus, where it regulates gene expression. GR activates or represses transcription of target genes by direct GRE binding, by tethering itself to other transcription factors apart from DNA binding, or in a composite manner by both direct GRE binding and interactions with transcription factors bound to neighboring sites. NPC = Nuclear pore complex; BTM = basal transcription machinery; TBP = TATA-binding protein; nGRE = negative GRE; RE = response element.

of Ser-404 has been shown to impact transcriptional activity of GR by impairing both activation and repression of target genes. Differences in cofactor recruitment have been implicated in these impaired transcriptional effects due to phosphorylation at Ser-404. Recently, our laboratory has identified a new hormone independent phosphorylation site Ser134. Serine 134 is hyperphosphorylated under an array of stressful conditions, including glucose starvation, oxidative stress, UV irradiation and osmotic shock. Phosphorylation of Ser-134 significantly increased the association of the GR with the ζ-isoform of the 14-3-3 class of signaling proteins (14-3-3ζ) on promoter proximal regions, resulting in a blunted hormone-dependent transcriptional response of specific genes. This study shows the level of molecular stress, as measured by Ser134-GR phosphorylation, has a global impact on the function of the signaling property of GR within animal cells [10].

GR is also subject to a variety of other posttranslational modifications. GR is ubiquitinated at a conserved lysine residue located in a PEST degradation motif, and this modification targets the receptor for degradation by the 26S proteasome. Mutation of this conserved Lys residue enhances the glucocorticoid-induced transcriptional activity of GR 4-fold and blocks ligand-dependent degradation of GR [11]. Another important posttranslational modification of GR is the covalent addition of a small ubiquitin-related modifier-1 (SUMO-1) termed sumoylation. GR is sumoylated at residues Lys-277, Lys-293 and Lys-703 [4]. Sumoylation of GRα has been shown to promote its degradation and inhibits the transcriptional activity of GR in a promoter-specific manner by recruiting corepressors.

Transcriptional Repression by the Glucocorticoid Receptor

Ligand-bound GR can repress target gene transcription by binding directly to DNA or by binding to other transcription factors. The former mechanism involves the binding of GR to less well-defined glucocorticoid-responsive elements called nGREs. It has been suggested that the GR functions passively at these nGRE by hampering the assembly of an activating transcription complex or the RNA polymerase. Recently, Surjit et al. [12] have shown that GR can actively repress target gene transcription by recruiting corepressors. They have identified yet another class of DNA response elements which contain inverted repeats of the sequence CTCC separated by either zero, one or two nucleotides. These novel nGREs have been shown to recruit NCoR1 and SMRT, which in turn engage HDACs to repress target gene transcription. This active repression mechanism has been linked to glucocorticoid effects on metabolism and bone [12]. However, few inflammatory genes that are repressed by glucocorticoids have been reported to utilize these nGREs, and further research will likely be necessary to define their role in this process.

Most of the anti-inflammatory effects of glucocorticoids appear to result from an important negative regulatory mechanism called transrepression, in which ligand-bound GR is recruited to chromatin by protein-protein interactions with DNA-bound transcription factors, particularly NF-κB and activator protein-1 (AP-1). It has been shown that transrepression requires the DBD of GR, but it does not depend on direct DNA binding. Repression is also accomplished on some genes by binding both a GRE and a transcription factor bound adjacent to the GRE in a composite manner [13]. The mechanism of transcriptional regulation by GR is complex (fig. 2). Operating through these diverse mechanisms, GR has been shown by microarray analysis to regulate up to 10–20% of the human genome in different cell types. Thus, when considering the transcriptional responses mediated by GR, one should take into account the absolute and relative abundance of the GR isoforms in different tissues, the location, accessibility and architecture of GREs as a function of chromatin landscape, the level of expression and activation of transcription factors with which GR associates, and the expression and availability of coregulators. Moreover, positive or negative regulatory activity appears likely to be dictated not simply by GR-binding site sequence but by chromatin context and by other transcription factors that bind in the vicinity of GR.

Mechanisms Contributing to Glucocorticoid Resistance

The anti-inflammatory and immunosuppressive effects of glucocorticoids are exploited extensively for the treatment of many inflammatory conditions. Due to the chronic nature of the inflammatory conditions, the treatment paradigms involve long-term glucocorticoid administration, which results in tolerance and induces the development of glucocorticoid resistance. Resistance to the therapeutic effects of glucocorticoids presents a considerable problem in managing these inflammatory diseases. In general, glucocorticoid resistance is defined as the inability of the cells to respond to all or a restricted number of glucocorticoid responses. At the molecular level, glucocorticoid resistance can be induced by several mechanisms and likely differs among patients. Glucocorticoid resistance can be attributed to reduced expression of GR, altered affinity of GR for the ligand, reduced ability of GR to bind DNA, or increased expression of inflammatory transcription factors like AP-1 that compete for DNA binding. Since resistance to glucocorticoids limits the therapeutic benefit of glucocorticoids, it is of clinical importance to elucidate molecular mechanisms of glucocorticoid resistance.

Polymorphisms and Somatic Mutations in the Glucocorticoid Receptor Gene

GR protein is the product of single gene located in chromosome 5 in humans. Somatic mutations in the gene are associated with specific types of disease, while numerous loss-of-function mutations in the GR gene have been observed in glucocorticoid-resistant human ALL cell lines. The combination of glucocorticoid and chemotherapy, with its mutagenic potential, might indeed favor the development of and subsequent selection for GR mutations. Hillman and colleagues showed that the glucocorticoid-resistant CCRF-CEM cell line contains one GR allele with the L753F mutation [14]. The LBD mutation (Δ702) of GR observed in glucocorticoid-resistant ALL patients emerged as the dominant population at relapse. Since the conventional assays for detection of aberrant GR mutations are inadequate in a heterogeneous cell population, GR mutations in patients are underrepresented as a mechanism of glucocorticoid resistance.

A polymorphism is defined as an inheritable genetic germ line variant of a single locus (most frequently a single nucleotide variation) that is present in at least 1% of the population. Inactivating single nucleotide polymorphisms within the LBD or the DBD of the receptor, and a 4-bp deletion at the 3′ boundary of exon 6 of the gene, have been described in glucocorticoid-resistant patients. Most of these mutations were heterozygous, indicating that complete loss-of-function of the receptor is incompatible with life. Severe impairment of the transactivation function of GR was observed in the cases of R477H, I559N, V571A, and D641V mutations. Furthermore, the mutant receptors hGRα I559N, F737L, I747M and L773P exerted a dominant negative effect upon the wild-type receptor [15]. Dexamethasone binding studies showed a variable reduction in the affinity of the mutant receptors for the ligand, with the most severe reduction observed in the cases of I559N. The ER22/23EK polymorphism that occurs in ~3% of the population results in an arginine (R) to lysine (K) change at position 23 (R23K) within the N terminus (fig. 1c). ER22/23EK is associated with decreased GR transcriptional activity in reporter assays and decreased expression of endogenous glucocorticoid responsive genes when compared to wild-type GR. Russcher and colleagues have shown an association between the ER22/23EK polymorphism and increases in the ratio of GRα-A to GRα-B. Adult carriers of the ER22/23EK polymorphism were shown to have a lower tendency to develop impaired glucose tolerance, type 2 diabetes and cardiovascular disease [16].

The N363S polymorphism, located within exon 2, occurs in ~4% of individuals, results in modest increases in GR transcriptional activity, and is associated with generalized increases in glucocorticoid sensitivity. Interestingly, microarray analysis revealed a unique polymorphism-specific pattern of gene regulation for N363S when compared to wild-type GRα. Furthermore, some studies associate N363S with an increased body mass index, coronary artery disease and decreased bone mineral density [17].

The A3669G polymorphism that is located within the 3′ untranslated region of GRβ results in increased stability of GRβ mRNA and the enhanced expression of GRβ protein (fig. 1c) [18]. Interestingly, A3669G is less capable of transrepressing the NFκB-regulated gene IL-2 than wild-type GRβ. Moreover, A3669G is associated with reduced immunosuppression. Individuals harboring A3669G have a higher incidence of rheumatoid arthritis and cardiovascular disease. Homozygous carriers of A3669G are associated with a proinflammatory phenotype that included an increased risk of myocardial infarction and coronary heart disease [16]. However, the spectrum of clinical manifestations in patients with GR mutations is quite broad, as a large number of subjects are asymptomatic and show only biochemical changes. Although the impact of GR polymorphisms and altered chaperone or cochaperone expression on glucocorticoid responsiveness in hematological malignancies is not well established, GR polymorphisms are emerging as an important biomarker for diseases of metabolic origin.

Glucocorticoid Receptor Expression Level

It is well documented that the level of GR protein determines the magnitude of glucocorticoid response. Several studies have shown that decreased GR expression in primary ALL cells is associated with initial resistance to glucocorticoid therapy, relapse and poor prognosis. GR levels in cells are dynamic, and are regulated in a cell type-specific manner by the surrounding concentration of ligand. In different cell lines and tissues, ligand induces downregulation of both GR mRNA and protein. Glucocorticoid-induced downregulation of GR mRNA has been attributed to reduce transcription of the GR gene as well as decreased stability of the GR mRNA [18, 19]. Previous studies from our laboratory have shown that the ligand-mediated downregulation of GR mRNA is mediated through the exonic region on the GR gene [20]. Additionally, proteosome-mediated degradation contributes to increased turnover of the GR protein in a ligand-dependent manner [11, 21]. Since GR can be ubiquitinated and tagged for proteasomal degradation, proteasome inhibitors might increase glucocorticoid responsiveness. However, this has not yet been shown in glucocorticoid-resistant disease. While hormone-induced downregulation of GR represents a mechanism for maintaining glucocorticoid homeostasis in normal cells, it has the potential to limit therapeutic responses to glucocorticoids in malignant cells. On the contrary, ligand induced upregulation of GR in lymphocytes is associated with glucocorticoid sensitivity. Thus, T cell lines that fail to auto-induce GR are resistant to glucocorticoid-induced apoptosis. Taken together, these findings suggest that GR expression level may be an important determinant of the glucocorticoid response [16]. The mechanisms underlying these processes are poorly understood, and further research is required to dissect their contribution to glucocorticoid resistance.

Glucocorticoid Receptor Heterogeneity

Glucocorticoid Receptor Isoforms Generated by Alternative Splicing

The α-isoform is the functional receptor and is encoded for by exons 2–9α. It is located in the cytoplasm in the absence of ligand, but translocates to the nucleus upon glucocorticoid binding. Alternative splicing of the GR primary transcript has been shown to generate a variant termed GRβ, a shorter protein with 742 residues. GRβ does not bind glucocorticoids, resides constitutively in the nucleus of cells, and does not directly regulate glucocorticoid-responsive reporter genes. However, when coexpressed with GRα, the splice variant functions as a dominant-negative inhibitor of GRα on genes both positively and negatively regulated by glucocorticoids. Various mechanisms, including competition for GRE binding, competition for transcriptional coregulators and formation of inactive GRα/GRβ heterodimers, have been proposed to underlie the antagonism [22]. Recent data show that GRβ, when introduced into cells in the absence GRα, does bind the synthetic GRα antagonist RU-486. In many cells and tissues examined, GRβ is expressed at low levels when compared to GRα, and in vitro studies have indicated that reductions in the cellular GRα:GRβ ratio contribute to glucocorticoid resistance. Resistance to glucocorticoid therapy in patients with leukemia and other diseases has been associated with high cellular levels of GRβ when compared to GRα, but this relationship has not been observed in other studies [23]. However, an association has been shown between reduced GRα:GRβ ratio and mood disorders such as schizophrenia, bipolar and major depressive disorder. As mentioned earlier, polymorphisms in GRβ have been linked to increased risk of myocardial infarction and coronary heart disease [24]. Another important finding has been the discovery of GRβ in mouse (mGRβ). This arises from a distinct mechanism that employs alternative splice donor sites in the intron separating exons 8 and 9. The resulting GRβ isoform is similar in structure and functionality to human GRβ. In addition, mGRβ exhibits ubiquitous expression, nuclear localization, inability to bind glucocorticoid agonists and antagonism of GRα [25]. Although GRβ does not bind to glucocorticoid, it is transcriptionally active, and the GR antagonist mifepristone can bind to it [24]. The endogenous ligand for GRβ is currently unknown.

The γ-isoform of GR (GRγ) is a splice variant in which exon 4 is alternatively spliced to exon 3, thereby including 3 bp of the intron region resulting in an additional arginine residue. This isoform is expressed at 3.8–8.7% of total GR mRNA in different human tissues. Ray and colleagues reported that the biological activity of the γ-isoform is reduced to 50% of the wild-type receptor. Gerdes and colleagues reported preliminary results showing a possible role for the γ-isoform in poor prednisone response in childhood ALL [16]. GRγ expression is also associated with glucocorticoid resistance in small cell lung carcinoma cells and corticotroph adenomas. The GR-A variant has an excision of exons 5, 6 and 7, resulting in an in-frame juxtaposition of exon 8 to 4. Little information is known about the expression levels and function of this variant. GR-P is missing exons 8 and 9, which encode the C-terminal half of the LBD due to a failure to splice at the exon 7/8 boundary. The GR-P transcripts account for up to 10–20% of total GR mRNA [4]. This GR variant has been reported to be upregulated in a small group of hematological malignancies (ALL, non-Hodgkin's lymphoma and multiple myeloma).

Our laboratory has identified N-terminal GR isoforms that are generated by alternative translation initiation from a single GR mRNA species. Internal conserved AUG codons corresponding to methionines 27, 86, 90, 98, 316, 331 and 336 were identified as bona fide translation start sites, generating proteins that have been termed GRα-B, C1, C2, C3, D1, D2 and D3, respectively. All GRα translational isoforms are expressed in various tissues in rat and mouse, but differences in expression levels between tissues are noted. Since the translational isoforms differ only by the length of their N-terminus, all 8 isoforms exhibit a similar affinity for ligand and most undergo hormone-induced nuclear localization. The GRα-D3 variant is the exception in that it localizes to the nucleus and can bind certain GREs even in the absence of hormone. The GRα-C3 variant is the most transcriptionally active, whereas the GRα-D proteins were the least active in reporter assays. These data suggest that the glucocorticoid-induced transcriptional response reflects the composite actions of GRα isoforms and that the specific intracellular pool of GRα subtypes may determine cellular sensitivity to glucocorticoids [26].

Microarray analysis and functional study of the various GRα isoforms revealed that the expression of the more active GRα-C3 correlated with increased sensitivity to glucocorticoid-induced apoptosis, and expression of the relatively inactive GRα-D3 was associated with resistance to glucocorticoid-induced apoptosis in U2-OS osteosarcoma cells stably expressing the individual translational isoforms. A recent study from our laboratory has shown that GRα-D, unlike the other receptor isoforms, does not inhibit the activity of an NF-κB-responsive reporter gene and does not efficiently repress either the transcription or translation of the antiapoptotic genes Bcl-xL, cellular inhibitor of apoptosis protein 1 and survivin. The inability of GRα-D to downregulate the expression of these genes appears to be associated with a diminished interaction between GRα-D and NF-κB. Thus, the D-isoform fails to interact with NF-κB in cells and promote apoptosis in response to glucocorticoids [27]. These data suggest that the N-terminal translational isoforms of GRα selectively regulate antiapoptotic genes and that the GRα-D isoform may contribute to the resistance of certain cancer cells to glucocorticoid-induced apoptosis. Genetic manipulation of the GR translational isoforms in animal models may shed new light on the biological importance of these intriguing GR variants, and it will be important to determine the contributions of a single GR isoform in whole animal. Furthermore, it is critical to verify if glucocorticoid-resistant cells exhibit an altered pattern of GR isoform expression.

Other Mechanisms of Glucocorticoid Resistance

Insufficient intracellular level of biologically active glucocorticoid is also responsible for glucocorticoid resistance. Insufficient levels of glucocorticoids may result from impaired uptake (regulated by P glycoprotein, multidrug resistance-associated protein, lung-resistance protein), increased steroid-binding proteins in the circulation or reduced converting enzyme activity (11β-hydroxysteroid dehydrogenase type 2) [16]. Nuclear translocation of GR is an important determinant of glucocorticoid sensitivity. Phosphorylation modulates the cellular trafficking of the receptor as GRα phosphorylated on Ser-203 is preferentially retained in the cytoplasm. A large proportion of patients with glucocorticoid-resistant asthma showed reduced nuclear translocation of GR and reduced GRE binding in PBMCs after glucocorticoid exposure, and this might be explained by GR phosphorylation [9, 23]. Since the mature GR heterocomplex is required for optimal ligand binding and subsequent activation of the transcriptional response, abnormalities in the chaperones and cochaperones that make up the heterocomplex may contribute to decreased glucocorticoid responsiveness. Kojika's group showed that alterations in hsp90 and hsp70 were associated with decreased cellular sensitivity [16]. Excessive activation of the transcription factors that GR interacts with has been identified as a mechanism of glucocorticoid resistance. Increased activation of AP1 has been recognized as a mechanism of glucocorticoid resistance in asthma, since this protein binds to GR and thus prevents its interaction with GRE and other transcription factors [23]. Furthermore, mutual antagonism between NF-κB and GR mediated by physical interaction (which is enhanced by CREB-binding protein) may be involved in decreased glucocorticoid sensitivity [28].

Conclusion

Glucocorticoids regulate numerous physiological processes, and are vital in the treatment of inflammation, autoimmune disease and cancer. The chronic nature of many of the inflammatory conditions and treatment paradigms frequently results in glucocorticoid resistance. Technological progress in molecular biology has advanced our understanding of the molecular mechanisms involved in glucocorticoid resistance, which includes reduced GR expression, GR downregulation, and acquired GR mutations. It is vital that our current understanding of these molecular mechanisms is translated into the clinic to aid in the development of safer and more effective glucocorticoid therapies.

Acknowledgements

We thank members of our laboratory for their critical reading of the manuscript. We thank NIEHS Arts and Photography for their help with the figures. This research was supported by the Intramural Research Program of the NIH, National Institute of Environmental Health Sciences.

References

1 Rhen T, Cidlowski JA: Antiinflammatory action of glucocorticoids – new mechanisms for old drugs. N Engl J Med 2005;353:1711–1723.

2 Schacke H, Hennekes H, Schottelius A, Jaroch S, Lehmann M, Schmees N, Rehwinkel H, Asadullah K: SEGRAS: a novel class of anti-inflammatory compounds. Ernst Schering Res Found Workshop 2002;357–371.

3 Clark AR, Belvisi MG: Maps and legends: the quest for dissociated ligands of the glucocorticoid receptor. Pharmacol Ther 2012;134:54–67.

4 Oakley RH, Cidlowski JA: Cellular processing of the glucocorticoid receptor gene and protein: new mechanisms for generating tissue-specific actions of glucocorticoids. J Biol Chem 2011;286:3177–3184.

5 Yudt MR, Cidlowski JA: Molecular identification and characterization of a and b forms of the glucocorticoid receptor. Mol Endocrinol 2001;15:1093–1103.

6 Lu NZ, Cidlowski JA: Translational regulatory mechanisms generate n-terminal glucocorticoid receptor isoforms with unique transcriptional target genes. Mol Cell 2005;18:331–342.

7 Biddie SC, Conway-Campbell BL, Lightman SL: Dynamic regulation of glucocorticoid signalling in health and disease. Rheumatology (Oxford) 2012; 51:403–412.

8 Reddy TE, Pauli F, Sprouse RO, Neff NF, Newberry KM, Garabedian MJ, Myers RM: Genomic determination of the glucocorticoid response reveals unexpected mechanisms of gene regulation. Genome Res 2009;19:2163–2171.

9 Galliher-Beckley AJ, Cidlowski JA: Emerging roles of glucocorticoid receptor phosphorylation in modulating glucocorticoid hormone action in health and disease. IUBMB Life 2009;61:979–986.

10 Galliher-Beckley AJ, Williams JG, Cidlowski JA: Ligand-independent phosphorylation of the glucocorticoid receptor integrates cellular stress pathways with nuclear receptor signaling. Mol Cell Biol 2011;31:4663–4675.

11 Wallace AD, Cidlowski JA: Proteasome-mediated glucocorticoid receptor degradation restricts transcriptional signaling by glucocorticoids. J Biol Chem 2001;276:42714–42721.

12 Surjit M, Ganti KP, Mukherji A, Ye T, Hua G, Metzger D, Li M, Chambon P: Widespread negative response elements mediate direct repression by agonist-liganded glucocorticoid receptor. Cell 2011; 145:224–241.

13 Barnes PJ: Anti-inflammatory actions of glucocorticoids: molecular mechanisms. Clin Sci (Lond) 1998;94:557–572.

14 Tissing WJ, Meijerink JP, den Boer ML, Pieters R: Molecular determinants of glucocorticoid sensitivity and resistance in acute lymphoblastic leukemia. Leukemia 2003;17:17–25.

15 Charmandari E, Kino T, Souvatzoglou E, Vottero A, Bhattacharyya N, Chrousos GP: Natural glucocorticoid receptor mutants causing generalized glucocorticoid resistance: molecular genotype, genetic transmission, and clinical phenotype. J Clin Endocrinol Metab 2004;89:1939–1949.

16 Gross KL, Lu NZ, Cidlowski JA: Molecular mechanisms regulating glucocorticoid sensitivity and resistance. Mol Cell Endocrinol 2009;300:7–16.

17 Jewell CM, Cidlowski JA: Molecular evidence for a link between the N363S glucocorticoid receptor polymorphism and altered gene expression. J Clin Endocrinol Metab 2007;92:3268–3277.

18 Schaaf MJ, Cidlowski JA: AUUUA motifs in the 3′UTR of human glucocorticoid receptor alpha and beta mRNA destabilize mRNA and decrease receptor protein expression. Steroids 2002;67:627–636.

19 Burnstein KL, Jewell CM, Cidlowski JA: Human glucocorticoid receptor cDNA contains sequences sufficient for receptor down-regulation. J Biol Chem 1990;265:7284–7291.

20 Burnstein KL, Jewell CM, Sar M, Cidlowski JA: Intragenic sequences of the human glucocorticoid receptor complementary DNA mediate hormone-inducible receptor messenger RNA down-regulation through multiple mechanisms. Mol Endocrinol 1994;8:1764–1773.

21 Wallace AD, Cao Y, Chandramouleeswaran S, Cidlowski JA: Lysine 419 targets human glucocorticoid receptor for proteasomal degradation. Steroids 2010;75:1016–1023.

22 Oakley RH, Jewell CM, Yudt MR, Bofetiado DM, Cidlowski JA: The dominant negative activity of the human glucocorticoid receptor beta isoform. Specificity and mechanisms of action. J Biol Chem 1999;274:27857–27866.

23 Barnes PJ: Mechanisms and resistance in glucocorticoid control of inflammation. J Steroid Biochem Mol Biol 2010;120:76–85.

24 Lewis-Tuffin LJ, Cidlowski JA: The physiology of human glucocorticoid receptor beta (HGRbeta) and glucocorticoid resistance. Ann N Y Acad Sci 2006;1069:1–9.

25 Hinds TD Jr, Ramakrishnan S, Cash HA, Stechschulte LA, Heinrich G, Najjar SM, Sanchez ER: Discovery of glucocorticoid receptor-beta in mice with a role in metabolism. Mol Endocrinol 2010;24:1715–1727.
26 Lu NZ, Collins JB, Grissom SF, Cidlowski JA: Selective regulation of bone cell apoptosis by translational isoforms of the glucocorticoid receptor. Mol Cell Biol 2007;27:7143–7160.
27 Gross KL, Oakley RH, Scoltock AB, Jewell CM, Cidlowski JA: Glucocorticoid receptor alpha isoform-selective regulation of antiapoptotic genes in osteosarcoma cells: a new mechanism for glucocorticoid resistance. Mol Endocrinol 2011;25:1087–1099.
28 McKay LI, Cidlowski JA: Cross-talk between nuclear factor-kappa b and the steroid hormone receptors: mechanisms of mutual antagonism. Mol Endocrinol 1998;12:45–56.

John A. Cidlowski
Laboratory of Signal Transduction, National Institute of Environmental Health Sciences
National Institutes of Health, Department of Health and Human Services
111 T.W. Alexander Dr., MD F3-07, Research Triangle Park, NC 27709 (USA)
E-Mail cidlows1@niehs.nih.gov

Maghnie M, Loche S, Cappa M, Ghizzoni L, Lorini R (eds): Hormone Resistance and Hypersensitivity. From Genetics to Clinical Management. Endocr Dev. Basel, Karger, 2013, vol 24, pp 57–66 (DOI: 10.1159/000342504)

ACTH Resistance: Genes and Mechanisms

E. Meimaridou · C.R. Hughes · J. Kowalczyk · L.F. Chan · A.J.L. Clark · L.A. Metherell

Centre for Endocrinology, William Harvey Research Institute, Barts and the London School of Medicine and Dentistry, Queen Mary University of London, London, UK

Abstract

ACTH resistance is a rare disorder typified by familial glucocorticoid deficiency (FGD), a genetically heterogeneous disease. Previously, genetic defects in FGD have been identified in the ACTH receptor gene *(MC2R)*, its accessory protein *(MRAP)* and the steroidogenic acute regulatory protein gene *(STAR)*. The defective mechanisms here are failures in ACTH ligand binding and/or receptor trafficking for MC2R and MRAP and, in the case of STAR mutations, inefficient cholesterol transport to allow steroidogenesis to proceed. Novel gene defects in FGD have recently been recognised in minichromosome maintenance-deficient 4 homologue (MCM4) and nicotinamide nucleotide transhydrogenase (NNT). MCM4 is one part of a DNA repair complex essential for DNA replication and genome stability, whilst NNT is involved in the glutathione redox system that protects cells against reactive oxygen species. The finding of mutations in these two genes implicates new pathogenetic mechanisms at play in FGD, and implies that the adrenal cortex is exquisitely sensitive to replicative and oxidative stresses.

Familial glucocorticoid deficiency (FGD) is a disease of ACTH resistance in which the cells of the zona fasciculata within the adrenal cortex fail to respond appropriately to stimulation by ACTH to produce cortisol [1]. The disease is characterised by glucocorticoid deficiency alone, and patients therefore exhibit low, often undetectable cortisol levels in concert with high ACTH levels. Patients typically present with symptoms related to their low cortisol and high ACTH [1]. Lack of glucocorticoids leads to hypoglycaemia and/or failure to thrive within the neonatal period or very early childhood; in older children the presentation may occur as a result of recurrent infections or hypoglycaemic seizures. If unrecognised/untreated, it can lead to learning difficulties secondary to recurrent hypoglycaemia or hypotension and neurological symptoms, and is potentially fatal. The excess ACTH often results in hyperpigmentation due to overstimulation of melanocortin 1 receptors (MC1R) [2]. This hyperpigmentation can be present from birth or may develop over time but is not always a feature; a notable exception was recently described in a Turkish child with FGD due to a homozygous MC2R mutation who had no excess pigmentation. The lack of pigmentation was due to the coexistence of a homozygous MC1R variant associated with red hair/fair skin [3]. Hence, the hyperpigmentation seen in FGD may be rarer in patients from white ethnicities where loss-of-function variants of MC1R are more common [3, 4].

Defects in the ACTH Receptor Pathway

Since this is a disorder of ACTH resistance, the first candidate gene was the ACTH receptor (melanocortin 2 receptor, MC2R, OMIM *607397). Mutations in this gene were discovered in 1993 in two siblings with FGD who had a homozygous base change causing substitution S74I [5]. Since that time, approximately 40 pathogenetic MC2R mutations have been reported throughout the world [1]. It quickly became obvious that the disease was genetically heterogeneous as MC2R mutations only accounted for about 25% of FGD patients [6]. It was also apparent that the expression of MC2R at the cell surface required an adrenal specific factor, since it proved difficult to express the receptor in cells that were not of adrenal origin. In order to search for this factor, a whole-genome scan by single nucleotide polymorphism (SNP) array genotyping in one consanguineous family was carried out and mapped a locus involved in FGD2 to chromosome 21q22.1 [7]. Screening for adrenal expression, by RT-PCR, of candidate genes within this region identified a single gene, melanocortin 2 receptor accessory protein (MRAP), as adrenal specific. Sequence analysis revealed a homozygous splice site mutation in the index family. Screening of the probands from a further 102 families with FGD type 2 identified a further five mutations (fig. 1). In total, 26 affected individuals from 21 families were identified, and therefore mutations in MRAP are responsible for a further 20% of FGD cases [7]. Since the first description, further mutations in MRAP have been described [8–11] including the first missense mutations, p.V26A and p.Y59D, which give rise to a milder, later onset form of the disease (fig. 1) [12].

Disease Mechanism for MC2R and MRAP Defects

MC2R is a seven-transmembrane G-protein-coupled receptor that binds its ligand, ACTH, at the cell surface; MRAP is a small single transmembrane accessory protein that forms an anti-parallel homodimer and is necessary to facilitate MC2R trafficking from the endoplasmic reticulum to the cell surface [13]. The underlying pathogenetic mechanism for these two causes of FGD is a failure of ACTH signalling either due to ineffective ligand binding or failure of trafficking of the receptor to the cell surface.

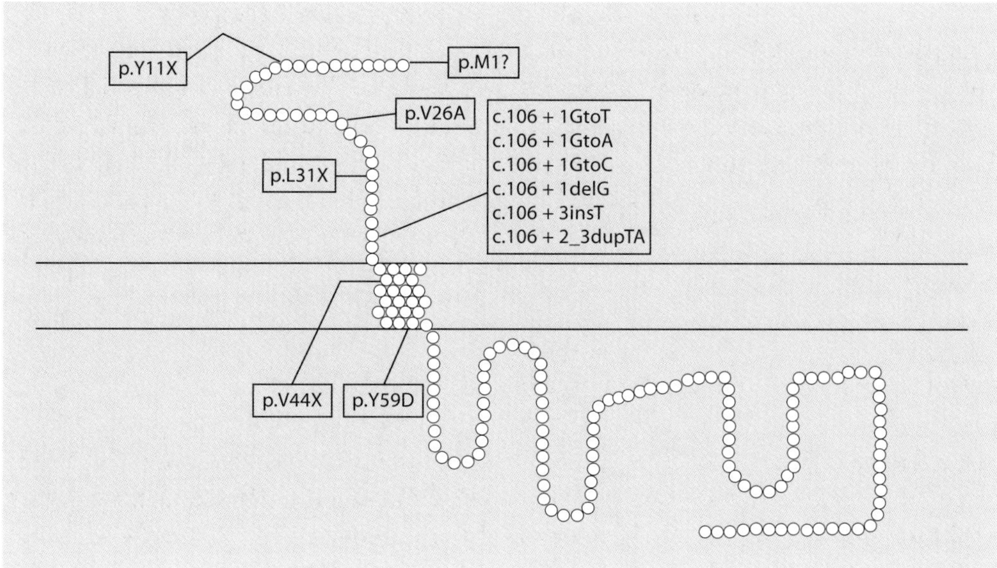

Fig. 1. Mutations in the *MRAP*. Cartoon depicting the protein structure of the single transmembrane domain MRAP protein. Mutations are represented at either protein level (denoted p.) or cDNA level (denoted c.). With the exception of p.Y59D and p.V26A, the two missense mutations, all the mutations will lead to early truncation of the protein and absence of the MC2R interacting transmembrane domain.

Most mutant MC2R proteins are trafficking defective, but in a few instances mutant MC2Rs fail to bind ACTH [14]. Apart from the recently described missense mutations, all MRAP mutations result in proteins lacking the transmembrane domain which is the MC2R interacting domain, and are therefore loss-of-function mutants causing ER retention of MC2R. The missense mutations have reduced functionality, but are trafficking competent, implying a probable signalling defect [12].

Defects in the Steroidogenic Pathway

Prior to the finding of mutations in MRAP in FGD, a region on chromosome 8q had been linked, by microsatellite analysis, to the disease in 3 families [6]. Reanalysis of this region by SNP genotyping was carried out in one of the three original 8q-linked families in the expectation of narrowing the size of the critical region and perhaps enabling a focused sequencing strategy [15]. In fact, this resulted in enlargement of the critical region enabling the identification of the steroidogenic acute regulatory protein (STAR) as a candidate. Sequencing revealed the index family had a homozygous R192C change in STAR, and 4 other families were found to have R188C mutations (fig. 2) [15]. More than 40 mutations in STAR have previously been described

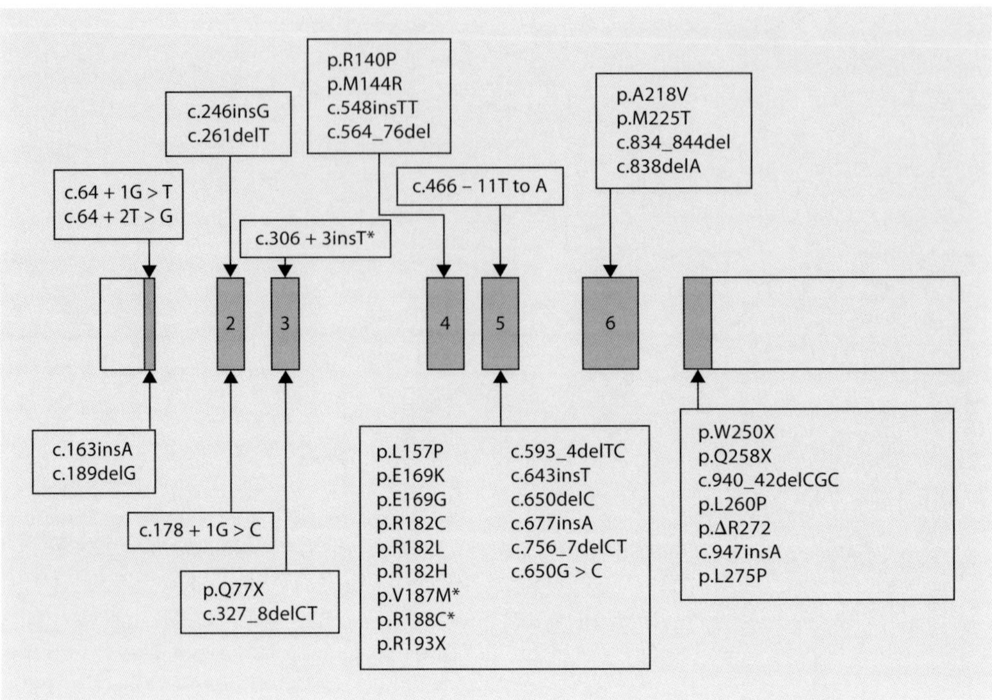

Fig. 2. Mutations in the *STAR*. Gene structure of *STAR* with mutations in each exon indicated in boxes. The mutations are described at either protein level (denoted p.) or cDNA level (denoted c.). Numbering is based on that given in the original manuscripts describing the mutations. Asterisk indicates 'mild' *STAR* mutations presenting with a FGD-like phenotype.

[16], mostly concentrated in the C-terminal half of the protein encoded by exons 5, 6, and 7 and causing lipoid congenital adrenal hyperplasia (OMIM, online mendelian inheritance in man, No. 201701). Patients with this condition usually present with a more severe phenotype than FGD exhibiting both adrenal and gonadal insufficiency, manifesting with high ACTH and renin levels coupled with low cortisol and aldosterone levels. In patients with a 46,XY karyotype, the absence of fetal testosterone/dihydrotestosterone production may lead to failure of androgenization and a female phenotype. Affected females undergo a normal puberty but have progressive hypergonadotropic hypogonadism.

Disease Mechanism for STAR Defects

STAR is responsible for the transfer of cholesterol across the mitochondrial membrane for the initial step of steroidogenesis, the conversion of cholesterol to pregnenolone, to occur (fig. 3). The failure of this and consequent build-up of cholesterol

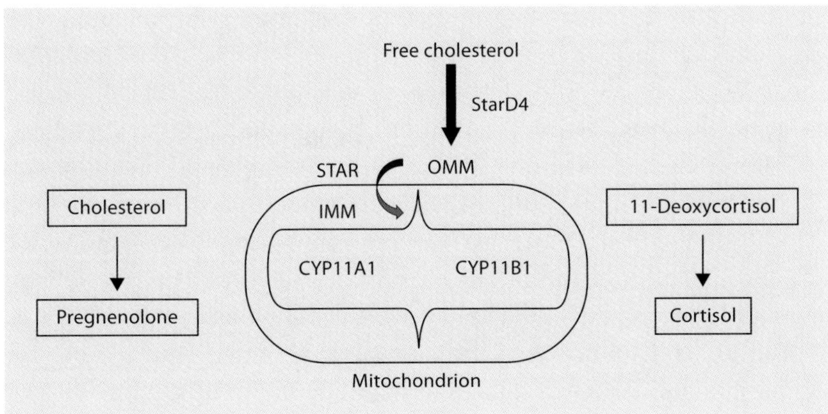

Fig. 3. Cholesterol delivery and mitochondrial steroidogenesis. Free cholesterol is delivered to the outer mitochondrial membrane (OMM) by StarD4 and transferred to the inner mitochondrial membrane (IMM) by STAR, where steroidogenesis begins. The first step of cortisol synthesis is the conversion of cholesterol to pregnenolone by CYP11A1 (side chain cleavage enzyme), and the last step is the conversion of 11-deoxycortisol to cortisol by CYP11B1; the steps in between occur outside the mitochondrion.

that results leads to steroidogenic cell destruction; hence, it is unsurprising that its loss leads to the phenotype seen in lipoid congenital adrenal hyperplasia. Most STAR mutations result in complete loss-of-function of the protein, whereas the R188C and R192C mutants retain >20% activity [17]. This may be the reason that patients with these mutations presented with a 'milder' phenotype and highlights the fact that patients with partially inactivating mutations in STAR can present a clinical phenotype that is compatible with a diagnosis of FGD [15, 17–19]. Such cases are more common than previously recognised, and account for up to 5% of our FGD cohort. The relative preservation of mineralocorticoid production probably reflects the lower production rate of aldosterone compared with cortisol which allows the adrenal zona glomerulosa to escape damage by lipid deposition. Furthermore, gonadal function allowed for normal male and female pubertal development and even fertility in some patients [15]. Others have shown similar findings [17–18], and in addition two recent publications report FGD-like phenotypes in patients with partial loss-of-function mutations in CYP11A1, the side chain cleavage enzyme responsible for the first step in steroidogenesis, the conversion of cholesterol to pregnenolone (fig. 3) [20, 21].

Defects in Replication Pathways

There were many FGD patients (~50%) without mutations in MC2R, MRAP or STAR and showing no linkage to these gene loci, including a group of patients from the Irish travelling community who had a unique variant of FGD [22]. Like classical FGD, affected children developed hypocortisolaemia and compensatory elevated ACTH, but retained normal renin and aldosterone levels. Unlike other forms of FGD, cortisol deficiency was not as pronounced, and onset was usually in childhood following a period of normal adrenal function [23]. In addition, in this unique form of the disorder patients had short stature, evidence of increased chromosomal breakage and natural killer cell deficiency [22, 23]. Autozygosity mapping in 8 affected children from 3 kindreds localised the disease locus to the pericentric region on chromosome 8. Targeted exome capture and high throughput sequencing identified the causal variant, c.71–1insG, in mini-chromosome maintenance-deficient 4 homologue (MCM4). This variant, a splice site mutation, led to the incorporation of an extra G into the mRNA, and was predicted to result in a foreshortened open reading frame encoding a prematurely terminated translation product (p.Pro24ArgfsX4). This mutation is believed to be unique to the Irish Traveller population.

Disease Mechanism for MCM4 Defect

MCM4 is one part of a heterohexameric complex (MCM2–7) responsible for normal DNA replication and genome stability in all eukaryotes; defects in MCM2–7 can cause genomic instability, leading to cancer and developmental defects in mice [24]. Given the essential role MCM4 plays in cell division, it was surprising that this mutation, causing early termination of the reading frame, should produce such a mild phenotype when gene knockout in mice is embryonic lethal [24]. Immunoblotting of patient lymphocytes showed loss of the full-length 96-kDa MCM4 protein as predicted from RNA analysis but showed evidence of a smaller, 85-kDa, MCM4 isoform [23]. The 85-kDa product was translated from an alternative initiation site downstream of the canonical ATG, and retained all the functional domains of the full-length product, which might explain the relatively mild phenotype in these patients compared to KO mice [23, 24]. Adrenals from an MCM4 depletion mouse model had abnormal morphology characterised by small, tightly packed, intensely stained spindle-shaped cells in the cortex; these cells were negative for CYP11A1 (P450 side chain cleavage) and CYP11B1 (P450 11β-hydroxylase), implying they were not capable of producing glucocorticoid. This abnormal adrenal morphology with steroidogenic cells displaced by non-steroidogenic cells, if recapitulated in the patients, is likely to compromise adrenal steroidogenesis.

Defects in Antioxidant Pathways

Linkage to a further locus on chromosome 5 was identified in 3 consanguineous families by SNP genotyping. Targeted exome sequencing of the proband from one 5-linked kindred identified a variant (c.1598C>T;p.Ala533Val) in nicotinamide

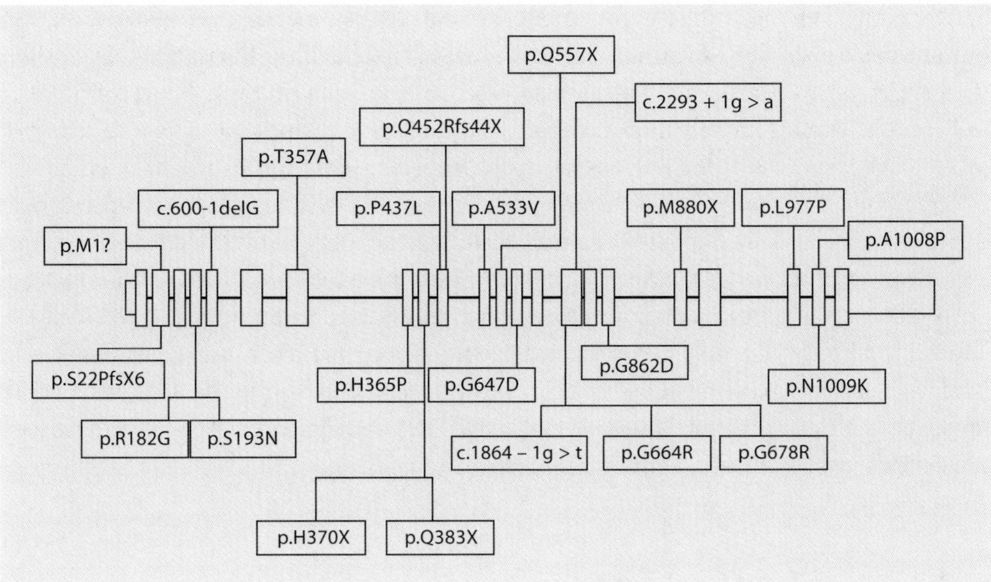

Fig. 4. Mutations in *NNT*. Cartoon depicting gene structure of *NNT* and the mutations described to date. Mutations are represented at either protein level (denoted p.) or cDNA level (denoted c.).

nucleotide transhydrogenase (NNT) as causal. Homozygous NNT mutations were also discovered in the two other chromosome 5-linked families, and 18 further mutations in 12 kindreds were found in homozygosity or compound heterozygosity on sequencing of 100 patients with FGD of unknown cause (fig. 4) [25]. These mutations were spread throughout the gene and included abolition of the initiating methionine, two further splice mutations and many missense and non-sense changes.

Disease Mechanism for Nicotinamide Nucleotide Transhydrogenase Defects

NNT, a highly conserved gene, encodes an integral protein of the inner mitochondrial membrane. Under most physiological conditions, this enzyme uses energy from the mitochondrial proton gradient to produce high concentrations of NADPH. Detoxification in mitochondria of reactive oxygen species (ROS) by glutathione peroxidases depends on this NADPH for regeneration of reduced glutathione (GSH) from oxidised glutathione (GSSG) to maintain a high GSH/GSSG ratio.

Adrenals from a C57BL6/J substrain of mice carrying a spontaneous Nnt mutation had slightly disorganised zonae fasciculata with higher levels of apoptosis than wild-type C57BL6/NHsd mice. Although there were no observable differences between the levels of CYP11A1 and CYP11B1 between the two substrains, the mutant mice did have lower basal and stimulated levels of corticosterone than their wild-type counterparts. Knockdown of NNT in the human adrenocortical H295R cell line by shRNA not only increased levels of mitochondrial ROS and apoptosis but also lowered the GSH/GSSG ratio, implying that NNT ablation causes an impairment of redox potential [25]. Oxidative stress has also been implicated in the pathogenesis of the closely related triple A syndrome (OMIM 231550). In this condition, mutations in AAAS lead to deficiency or mislocalization of the nuclear-pore protein ALADIN resulting in impairment of the nuclear import of DNA repair and antioxidant proteins, thereby rendering the patients' cells more susceptible to oxidative stress. The finding of NNT mutations in FGD suggests that, at least in humans, NNT is of primary importance for ROS detoxification in adrenocortical cells, highlighting the susceptibility of the adrenal cortex to this type of pathological damage.

Conclusion

Historically, defects in the ACTH receptor pathway, MC2R and its accessory protein MRAP, were known to cause FGD. More recently, partial loss-of-function mutations in steroidogenic pathway genes, STAR and CYP11A1, have been recognised as causal. The discovery of defects in DNA replication and antioxidant genes, MCM4 and NNT, expands the spectrum of pathways that can be pathogenic in ACTH resistance. Exactly why these gene defects should preferentially affect the adrenal production of hormones is not known, but is currently under investigation. The finding of mutations in these two genes implies that the adrenal cortex is exquisitely sensitive to replicative and oxidative stresses. Over time, patients with MCM4 or NNT mutations may develop other organ pathologies related to their impaired gene functions, and will therefore need careful monitoring.

References

1 Clark AJ, Chan LF, Chung TT, Metherell LA: The genetics of familial glucocorticoid deficiency. Best Pract Res Clin Endocrinol Metab 2009;23:159–165.

2 Chung TT, Chan LF, Metherell LA, Clark AJ: Phenotypic characteristics of familial glucocorticoid deficiency (FGD) type 1 and 2. Clin Endocrinol (Oxf) 2009;72:589–594.

3 Turan S, Hughes C, Atay Z, Guran T, Haliloglu B, Clark AJ, Bereket A, Metherell LA: An atypical case of familial glucocorticoid deficiency without pigmentation caused by coexistent homozygous mutations in MC2R (T152K) and MC1R (R160W). J Clin Endocrinol Metab 2012;97:E771–E774.

4 Smith R, Healy E, Siddiqui S, Flanagan N, Steijlen PM, Rosdahl I, Jacques JP, Rogers S, Turner R, Jackson IJ, Birch-Machin MA, Rees JL: Melanocortin 1 receptor variants in an Irish population. J Invest Dermatol 1998;111:119–122.
5 Clark AJ, McLoughlin L, Grossman A: Familial glucocorticoid deficiency associated with point mutation in the adrenocorticotropin receptor. Lancet 1993;341:461–462.
6 Génin E, Huebner A, Jaillard C, Faure A, Halaby G, Saka N, Clark AJ, Durand P, Bégeot M, Naville D: Linkage of one gene for familial glucocorticoid deficiency type 2 (FGD2) to chromosome 8q and further evidence of heterogeneity. Hum Genet 2002; 111:428–434.
7 Metherell LA, Chapple JP, Cooray S, David A, Becker C, Ruschendorf F, Naville D, Begeot M, Khoo B, Nurnberg P, Huebner A, Cheetham ME, Clark AJ: Mutations in MRAP, encoding a new interacting partner of the ACTH receptor, cause familial glucocorticoid deficiency type 2. Nat Genet 2005;37:166–170.
8 Modan-Moses D, Ben-Zeev B, Hoffmann C, Falik-Zaccai TC, Bental YA, Pinhas-Hamiel O, Anikster Y: Unusual presentation of familial glucocorticoid deficiency with a novel MRAP mutation. J Clin Endocrinol Metab 2006;91:3713–3717.
9 Rumié H, Metherell LA, Clark AJ, Beauloye V, Maes M: Clinical and biological phenotype of a patient with familial glucocorticoid deficiency type 2 caused by a mutation of melanocortin 2 receptor accessory protein. Eur J Endocrinol 2007;157:539–542.
10 Akın L, Kurtoğlu S, Kendirici M, Akın MA: Familial glucocorticoid deficiency type 2: a case report. J Clin Res Pediatr Endocrinol 2010;2:122–125.
11 Jain V, Metherell LA, David A, Sharma R, Sharma PK, Clark AJ, Chan LF: Neonatal presentation of familial glucocorticoid deficiency resulting from a novel splice mutation in the melanocortin 2 receptor accessory protein. Eur J Endocrinol 2011; 165:987–991.
12 Hughes CR, Chung TT, Habeb AM, Kelestimur F, Clark AJ, Metherell LA: Missense mutations in the melanocortin 2 receptor accessory protein that lead to late onset familial glucocorticoid deficiency type 2. J Clin Endocrinol Metab 2010;95:3497–3501.
13 Webb TR, Clark AJ: Minireview: the melanocortin 2 receptor accessory proteins. Mol Endocrinol 2010;24:475–484.
14 Chung TT, Webb TR, Chan LF, Cooray SN, Metherell LA, King PJ, Chapple JP, Clark AJ: The majority of adrenocorticotropin receptor (melanocortin 2 receptor) mutations found in familial glucocorticoid deficiency type 1 lead to defective trafficking of the receptor to the cell surface. J Clin Endocrinol Metab 2008;93:4948–4954.
15 Metherell LA, Naville D, Halaby G, Begeot M, Huebner A, Nürnberg G, Nürnberg P, Green J, Tomlinson JW, Krone NP, Lin L, Racine M, Berney DM, Achermann JC, Arlt W, Clark AJL: Non-classic lipoid congenital adrenal hyperplasia masquerading as familial glucocorticoid deficiency. J Clin Endocrinol Metab 2009;94:3865–3871.
16 Miller WL, Bose HS: Early steps in steroidogenesis: intracellular cholesterol trafficking. J Lipid Res 2011;52:2111–2135.
17 Baker BY, Lin L, Kim CJ, Raza J, Smith CP, Miller WL, Achermann JC: Nonclassic congenital lipoid adrenal hyperplasia: a new disorder of the steroidogenic acute regulatory protein with very late presentation and normal male genitalia. J Clin Endocrinol Metab 2006;91:4781–4785.
18 Flück CE, Pandey AV, Dick B, Camats N, Fernández-Cancio M, Clemente M, Gussinyé M, Carrascosa A, Mullis PE, Audi L: Characterization of novel StAR (steroidogenic acute regulatory protein) mutations causing non-classic lipoid adrenal hyperplasia. PLoS One 2011;6:e20178.
19 Sahakitrungruang T, Soccio RE, Lang-Muritano M, Walker JM, Achermann JC, Miller WL: Clinical, genetic, and functional characterization of four patients carrying partial loss-of-function mutations in the steroidogenic acute regulatory protein (StAR). J Clin Endocrinol Metab 2010;95:3352–3359.
20 Parajes S, Kamrath C, Rose IT, Taylor AE, Mooij CF, Dhir V, Grötzinger J, Arlt W, Krone N: A novel entity of clinically isolated adrenal insufficiency caused by a partially inactivating mutation of the gene encoding for P450 side chain cleavage enzyme (CYP11A1). J Clin Endocrinol Metab 2011;96:1798–1806.
21 Sahakitrungruang T, Tee MK, Blackett PR, Miller WL: Partial defect in the cholesterol side-chain cleavage enzyme P450scc (CYP11A1) resembling nonclassic congenital lipoid adrenal hyperplasia. J Clin Endocrinol Metab 2011;96:792–798.
22 O'Riordan SM, Lynch SA, Hindmarsh PC, Chan LF, Clark AJ, Costigan C: A novel variant of familial glucocorticoid deficiency prevalent among the Irish Traveler population. J Clin Endocrinol Metab 2008;93:2896–2899.

23 Hughes CR, Guasti L, Meimaridou E, Chuang CH, Schimenti JC, King PJ, Costigan C, Clark AJ, Metherell LA: MCM4 mutation causes adrenal failure, short stature, and natural killer cell deficiency in humans. J Clin Invest 2012;122:814–820.

24 Chuang CH, Wallace MD, Abratte C, Southard T, Schimenti JC: Incremental genetic perturbations to MCM2–7 expression and subcellular distribution reveal exquisite sensitivity of mice to DNA replication stress. PLoS Genet 2010;6:pii e1001110.

25 Meimaridou E, Kowalczyk J, Guasti L, Hughes CR, Wagner F, Frommolt P, Nürnberg P, Mann NP, Banerjee R, Saka HN, Chapple JP, King PJ, Clark AJL, Metherell LA: Mutations in NNT encoding nicotinamide nucleotide transhydrogenase cause familial glucocorticoid deficiency. Nat Genet 2012;44:740–742.

Lou Metherell
Centre for Endocrinology, William Harvey Research Institute
Barts and the London School of Medicine and Dentistry, Queen Mary University of London
EC1M 6BQ, London (UK)
E-Mail l.a.metherell@qmul.ac.uk

Maghnie M, Loche S, Cappa M, Ghizzoni L, Lorini R (eds): Hormone Resistance and Hypersensitivity. From Genetics to Clinical Management. Endocr Dev. Basel, Karger, 2013, vol 24, pp 67–85 (DOI: 10.1159/000342505)

Primary Generalized Familial and Sporadic Glucocorticoid Resistance (Chrousos Syndrome) and Hypersensitivity

Evangelia Charmandari[a–c] · Tomoshige Kino[c] · George P. Chrousos[a–c]

[a]Division of Endocrinology, Metabolism and Diabetes, First Department of Pediatrics, University of Athens Medical School, Aghia Sophia Children's Hospital, [b]Division of Endocrinology and Metabolism, Clinical Research Center, Biomedical Research Foundation of the Academy of Athens, Athens, Greece; [c]Unit on Molecular Hormone Action, Program in Reproductive and Adult Endocrinology, Eunice Kennedy Shriver National Institute of Child Health and Human Development, National Institutes of Health, Bethesda, Md., USA

Abstract

Familial or sporadic primary generalized glucocorticoid resistance or Chrousos syndrome is a rare genetic condition characterized by generalized, partial, target-tissue insensitivity to glucocorticoids and a consequent hyperactivation of the hypothalamic-pituitary-adrenal (HPA) axis. Primary generalized glucocorticoid hypersensitivity (PGGH) represents the mirror image of the former, and is characterized by generalized, partial, target-tissue hypersensitivity to glucocorticoids, and compensatory hypoactivation of the HPA axis. The molecular basis of both conditions has been ascribed to mutations in the human glucocorticoid receptor (hGR) gene, which impair the molecular mechanisms of hGR action and alter tissue sensitivity to glucocorticoids. This review summarizes the pathophysiology, molecular mechanisms and clinical aspects of Chrousos syndrome and PGGH.

In humans, glucocorticoids regulate a broad spectrum of physiologic functions essential for life, and play important roles in the maintenance of basal and stress-related homeostasis [1–4]. Glucocorticoids participate in almost every cellular, molecular and physiologic network of the organism, and play pivotal roles in critical biologic processes, such as growth, reproduction, intermediary metabolism, the immune and inflammatory reaction, as well as central nervous system and cardiovascular functions [1, 4]. In addition, glucocorticoids represent one of the most widely used therapeutic agents, often employed in the treatment of inflammatory, autoimmune and lymphoproliferative disorders [1].

The Human Glucocorticoid Receptor

At the cellular level, the actions of glucocorticoids are mediated by a 94-kDa protein, the glucocorticoid receptor (GR). The human GR (hGR) belongs to the steroid/thyroid/retinoic acid superfamily of nuclear receptors, and functions as a ligand-dependent transcription factor that regulates the expression of glucocorticoid-responsive genes positively or negatively [5–7] (fig. 1a). The hGR gene locus is on the long arm of chromosome 5 (q31.3) and consists of 9 exons. Alternative splicing of the hGR gene in exon 9 generates two highly homologous receptor isoforms, termed α and β. These are identical through amino acid 727, but then diverge, with hGRα having an additional 50 amino acids and hGRβ having an additional 15 nonhomologous amino acids [3, 5–8] (fig. 1a). The hGRα represents the classic GR that functions as a ligand-dependent transcription factor and mediates the classic actions of glucocorticoids. The hGRβ, on the other hand, does not bind glucocorticoid agonists, has intrinsic, hGRα-independent, gene-specific transcriptional activity, and exerts a dominant negative effect upon the transcriptional activity of hGRα [9, 10].

The hGR is a modular protein composed of distinct regions illustrated in figure 1b: the amino-terminal A/B region, also called immunogenic or N-terminal domain (NTD), and the C, D and E regions, which correspond to the DNA-binding domain (DBD), the hinge region and the ligand-binding domain (LBD), respectively [3, 5, 6].

Expressed hGRα is represented by a panel of 8 amino terminal translational isoforms of varying lengths. These hGRα isoforms differ at their amino-termini, cytoplasmic/nuclear distribution and cell-specific expression, and may differentially transduce the glucocorticoid signal in target tissues. It is likely that similar differential cell-specific production and functional differences might also be present between the 8 putative hGRβ translational isoforms [5, 6]. This marked complexity in the transcription/translation of the hGR gene enables target tissues to differentially respond to circulating glucocorticoid concentrations and accounts for the highly stochastic nature of the glucocorticoid signaling pathway [11].

In the absence of ligand, hGRα resides mostly in the cytoplasm of cells as part of a hetero-oligomeric complex, which contains chaperon heat shock proteins 90, 70 and FKBP51, as well as other proteins [7, 11]. Following ligand-induced activation, the hGRα dissociates from this multiprotein complex and translocates into the nucleus, where it binds as a homodimer to glucocorticoid response elements (GREs) in the promoter regions of target genes, and regulates their expression positively or negatively [7, 11] (fig. 2). To initiate transcription, the hGRα isoform(s) uses its transcriptional activation domains, activation function (AF)-1 and AF-2, located in the NTD and LBD, respectively, as surfaces to interact with nuclear receptor coactivators and chromatin-remodeling complexes [12–15]. The ligand-activated hGRα can also modulate gene expression independently of DNA binding, by interacting, possibly as a monomer, with other transcription factors, such as nuclear factor-κB, activator protein-1, p53 and signal transducers and activators of transcription [7]. Following

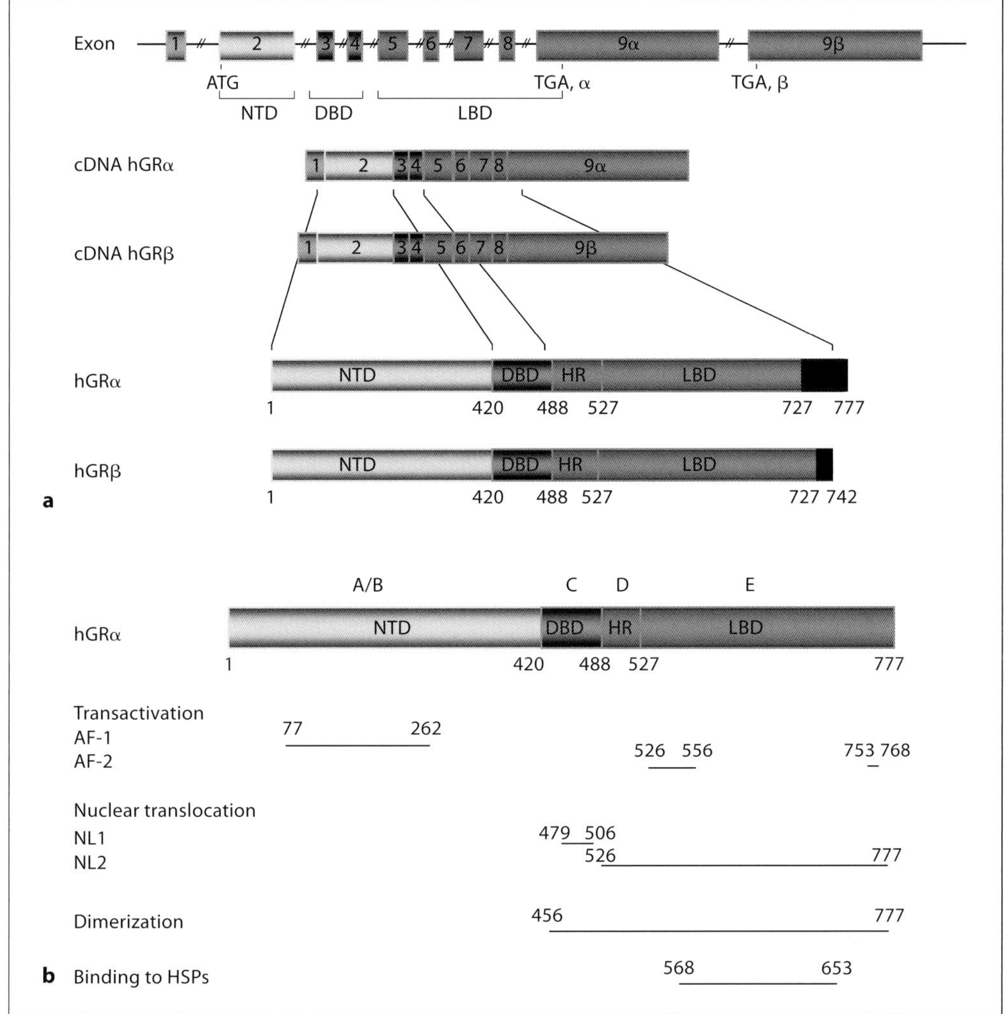

Fig. 1. **a** Schematic representation of the structure of the hGR gene. Alternative splicing of the primary transcript gives rise to the two mRNA and protein isoforms, hGRα and hGRβ. **b** Functional domains of the hGRα. The functional domains and subdomains are indicated beneath the linearized protein structures. NL = Nuclear localization.

transcriptional activation or inhibition of glucocorticoid-responsive genes, hGRα dissociates from the ligand, and has a lower affinity for binding to GREs located in their regulatory areas. The unliganded hGRα remains within the nucleus for a considerable length of time, and is then exported to the cytoplasm; both within the nucleus and within the cytoplasm, the hGRα may be recycled and/or degraded in the proteasomes [16] (fig. 2).

Alterations in the molecular mechanisms of hGRα action may lead to alterations in tissue sensitivity to glucocorticoids, which may take the form of *glucocorticoid*

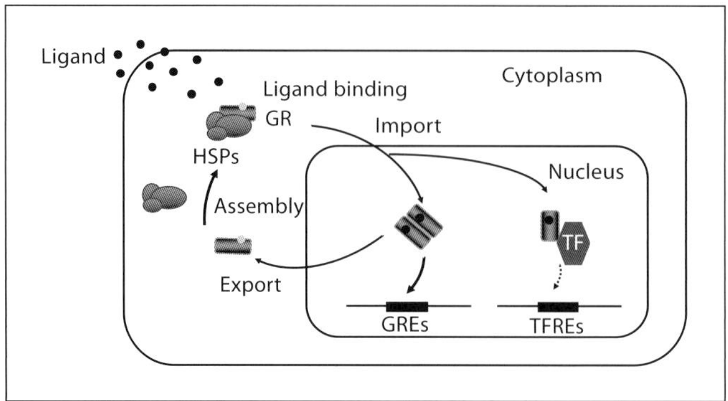

Fig. 2. Nucleocytoplasmic shuttling of the GR. Upon binding to the ligand, the activated hGRα dissociates from heat shock proteins (HSPs) and translocates into the nucleus, where it homodimerizes and binds to GREs in the promoter region of target genes or interacts with other transcription factors (TFs), such as activator protein-1, nuclear factor-κB and signal transducer and activator of transcription-5, ultimately modulating the transcriptional activity of respectively GRE- or TFRE-containing genes.

resistance or *glucocorticoid hypersensitivity* and may be associated with significant morbidity [17–19]. In the present review, we summarize the pathophysiology and molecular mechanisms underlying Chrousos syndrome and primary generalized glucocorticoid hypersensitivity (PGGH).

Chrousos Syndrome and Primary Generalized Glucocorticoid Hypersensitivity

Clinical Manifestations

Chrousos syndrome is a rare familial or sporadic condition characterized by generalized, mostly partial, target-tissue insensitivity to glucocorticoids, which leads to compensatory activation of the hypothalamic-pituitary-adrenal (HPA) axis and hypersecretion of adrenocorticotropic hormone (ACTH) in the systemic circulation [20–22]. The latter results in adrenocortical hyperplasia/hypertrophy, increased cortisol secretion as a compensation for the reduced action of glucocorticoids at the brain and pituitary negative feedback-regulated areas of the HPA axis and increased production of adrenal steroids with mineralocorticoid (cortisol, deoxycorticosterone and corticosterone) and/or androgenic activity [androstenedione, dehydroepiandrosterone (DHEA) and DHEA-sulfate (DHEAS)] [20–22].

The clinical manifestations of primary generalized glucocorticoid resistance (PGGR) reflect the pathophysiologic alterations described above, and primarily include those of mineralocorticoid and/or androgen excess; they are summarized in table 1 [20–22]. Clinical manifestations of glucocorticoid deficiency might occur, but are rare

Table 1. Clinical manifestations and diagnostic evaluation of generalized glucocorticoid resistance

Clinical presentation
Apparently normal glucocorticoid function
Asymptomatic
Chronic fatigue (glucocorticoid deficiency?)
Mineralocorticoid excess
Hypertension
Hypokalemic alkalosis
Androgen excess
Children: ambiguous genitalia at birth[1], premature adrenarche, precocious puberty
Females: acne, hirsutism, male-pattern hair loss, menstrual irregularities, oligoanovulation, infertility
Males: acne, hirsutism, oligospermia, adrenal rests in the testes, infertility
Increased HPA axis activity (CRH/ACTH hypersecretion)
Anxiety
Adrenal rests
Diagnostic evaluation
Absence of clinical features of Cushing syndrome
Normal or elevated plasma ACTH concentrations
Elevated plasma cortisol concentrations
Increased 24-hour UFC excretion
Normal circadian and stress-induced pattern of cortisol and ACTH secretion
Resistance of the HPA axis to dexamethasone suppression
Thymidine incorporation assays: increased resistance to dexamethasone-induced suppression of phytohemaglutinin-stimulated thymidine incorporation compared to control subjects
Dexamethasone-binding assays: decreased affinity of the GR for the ligand compared to control subjects
Molecular studies: mutations/deletions of the GR

Modified from Charmandari et al. [22].

[1] This is the only case of ambiguous genitalia documented in a child with 46,XX karyotype who also harbored a heterozygous mutation of the 21-hydroxylase gene.

and were only reported in a young child with hypoglycemic generalized tonic-clonic seizures during the course of a febrile illness [23], in a newborn baby with severe hypoglycemia, excessive 'fatigability' with feeding, increased susceptibility to infections and concurrent growth hormone deficiency [24], and in several adult patients with chronic fatigue [20–22]. The clinical spectrum of the condition is broad, ranging from most severe to mild or even asymptomatic forms [20–22]. This variable clinical phenotype is due to variations in the tissue sensitivity of the glucocorticoid, mineralocorticoid and/or androgen receptor signaling pathways, variations in the activity of key hormone-inactivating or -activating enzymes, such as the 11β-hydroxysteroid dehydrogenase [25] and other genetic or epigenetic factors, such as the presence of insulin resistance and visceral obesity [21]. It has been proposed that the term Chrousos syndrome is used in place of familial and sporadic PGGR [26, 27].

PGGH represents the mirror image of Chrousos syndrome, and is characterized by generalized, partial, target-tissue hypersensitivity to glucocorticoids, and compensatory hypoactivation of the HPA axis. To date, there has been only one patient reported with manifestations of tissue-specific glucocorticoid hypersensitivity caused by a novel hGR gene mutation. The patient was a 43-year-old female who presented with a long-standing history of visceral obesity, hypercholesterolemia, hypertriglyceridemia, diabetes type 2 and hypertension [28] (table 2).

Molecular Mechanisms

hGR Mutations

The molecular basis of Chrousos syndrome has been ascribed primarily to mutations in the hGR gene, which impair the molecular mechanisms of hGR action and decrease tissue sensitivity to glucocorticoids (table 2; fig. 3) [23, 24, 29–41]. The molecular defects that have been elucidated in cases with Chrousos syndrome and have been reported to date are summarized in table 2. We have identified most hGR mutations associated with PGGR and have systematically investigated the molecular mechanisms through which these various natural hGR mutants affect glucocorticoid signal transduction in almost all reported cases of generalized glucocorticoid resistance. We studied: (a) the transcriptional activity of the mutant receptors; (b) the ability of the mutant receptors to exert a dominant negative effect upon the wild-type receptor; (c) the affinity of the mutant receptors for the ligand; (d) the subcellular localization of the mutant receptors and their nuclear translocation following exposure to the ligand; (e) the ability of the mutant receptors to bind to GREs, and (f) the interaction of the mutant receptors with the GR-interacting protein-1 (GRIP1) coactivator, which belongs to the p160 family of nuclear receptor coactivators and plays an important role in the hGRα-mediated transactivation of glucocorticoid-responsive genes [22, 29–40].

Compared with the wild-type receptor, all mutant receptors demonstrated variable reduction in their ability to transactivate glucocorticoid-responsive genes in response to dexamethasone [29–40]. The mutant receptors hGRαI559N, hGRαF737L, hGRαI747M and hGRαL773P exerted a dominant negative effect upon the wild-type receptor, which might have contributed to manifestation of the disease at the heterozygote state [29, 33, 35, 37, 40]. All mutant receptors in which the mutations were located in the LBD of the receptor showed a variable reduction in their affinity for the ligand [29–40]. The mutant receptors that demonstrated normal affinity for the ligand were the hGRαR477H and hGRαV423A, in which the mutations were located in the DBD [39, and unpublished data]. Most pathologic mutant receptors were observed primarily in the cytoplasm of cells in the absence of ligand, except for the hGRαV729I and hGRαF737L receptors, which were localized both in the cytoplasm and the nucleus of cells. Exposure to dexamethasone induced a slow translocation of the

Table 2. Mutations of the hGR gene causing PGGR or hypersensitivity

Reference	Mutation position		Molecular mechanisms	Genotype	Phenotype
	cDNA	amino acid			
Chrousos et al. [20]	1922 (A→T)	641 (D→V)	transactivation ↓	homozygous	hypertension
Hurley et al. [30]			affinity for ligand ↓ (×3)		hypokalemic alkalosis
			nuclear translocation: 22 min		
			abnormal interaction with GRIP1		
Karl et al. [31]	4-bp deletion in exon-intron 6		hGRα number: 50% of control	heterozygous	hirsutism
			inactivation of the affected allele		male pattern hair-loss
					menstrual irregularities
Malchoff et al. [32]	2185 (G→A)	729 (V→I)	transactivation ↓	homozygous	precocious puberty
			affinity for ligand ↓ (×2)		hyperandrogenism
			nuclear translocation: 120 min		
			abnormal interaction with GRIP1		
Karl et al. [29]	1676 (T→A)	559 (I→N)	transactivation ↓	heterozygous	hypertension
Kino et al. [33]			decrease in hGR-binding sites		oligospermia
			transdominance (+)		infertility
			nuclear translocation: 180		
			abnormal interaction with GRIP1		
Ruiz et al. [34]	1430 (G→A)	477 (R→H)	transactivation ↓	heterozygous	hirsutism
Charmandari et al. [39]			no DNA binding		fatigue
			nuclear translocation: 20 min		hypertension
Ruiz et al. [34]	2035 (G→A)	679 (G→S)	transactivation ↓	heterozygous	hirsutism
Charmandari et al. [39]			affinity for ligand ↓ (×2)		fatigue
			nuclear translocation: 30 min		hypertension
			abnormal interaction with GRIP1		

Table 2. continued

Reference	Mutation position		Molecular mechanisms	Genotype	Phenotype
	cDNA	amino acid			
Mendonca et al. [35]	1712 (T→C)	571 (V→A)	transactivation ↓	homozygous	ambiguous genitalia
			affinity for ligand ↓ (×6)		hypertension
			nuclear translocation: 25 min		hypokalemia
			abnormal interaction with GRIP1		hyperandrogenism
Vottero et al. [36]	2241 (T→G)	747 (I→M)	transactivation ↓	heterozygous	cystic acne
			transdominance (+)		hirsutism
			affinity for ligand ↓ (×2)		oligoamenorrhea
			nuclear translocation ↓		
			abnormal interaction with GRIP1		
Charmandari et al. [38]	2318 (T→C)	773 (L→P)	transactivation ↓	heterozygous	fatigue
			transdominance (+)		anxiety
			affinity for ligand ↓ (×2.6)		acne
			nuclear translocation: 30 min		hirsutism
			abnormal interaction with GRIP1		hypertension
Charmandari et al. [40]	2209 (T→C)	737 (F→L)	transactivation ↓	heterozygous	hypertension
			transdominance (time-dependent) (+)		hypokalemia
			affinity for ligand ↓ (×1.5)		
			nuclear translocation: 180 min		
Nader et al. [23]	2141 (G→A)	714 (R→Q)	transactivation ↓	heterozygous	hypoglycemia
			transdominance (+)		hypokalemia
			affinity for ligand ↓ (×2)		hypertension
			nuclear translocation ↓		mild clitoromegaly
			abnormal interaction with GRIP1		advanced bone age
					precocious pubarche

Table 2. continued

Reference	Mutation position		Molecular mechanisms	Genotype	Phenotype
	cDNA	amino acid			
McMahon et al. [24]	2-bp deletion at nt 2318-9	773	transactivation ↓	homozygous	hypoglycemia
			affinity for ligand: absent		fatigability with feeding
			no suppression of IL-6		hypertension
Zhu et al. [41]	1667 (G→T)	556 (T→I)	not studied yet	heterozygous	adrenal incidentaloma
Charmandari et al. [28]	1201 (G→C)	401 (D→H)	transactivation ↑	heterozygous	visceral obesity
			transdominance (+)		hypercholesterolemia
			affinity for ligand: N		hypertriglyceridemia
			nuclear translocation: N		hypertension
			interaction with GRIP1: N		diabetes type 2

Modified from Chrousos et al. [20, 21] and Charmandari et al. [22].

mutant receptors into the nucleus, which ranged from 20 to 180 min compared with the wild-type hGRα, which required only 12 min for complete translocation [29–40]. All mutant receptors in which the mutations were located in the LBD preserved their ability to bind to DNA and displayed an abnormal interaction with the GRIP1 coactivator in vitro [29–40]. The mutant receptors that failed to bind to DNA or reduced the ability of the receptor to bind to DNA but displayed a normal interaction with the GRIP1 coactivator were the hGRαR477H and hGRαV423A, respectively, in which the mutation was localized in the DBD of the receptor, thus preserving the structure and function of both NTD and LBD and ensuring normal interaction with this coactivator [39, and unpublished data]. Since the binding of these receptors to DNA is followed by the attraction of GRIP1 coactivator to the transcriptional complex formed with GR on DNA, the normal interaction of hGRαR477H and hGRαV423A with GRIP1 would contribute minimally to the transcriptional activity induced by these receptors [39].

In the patient with the symptomatology suggestive of PGGH, we identified a novel, heterozygous guanine to cytosine (G→C) substitution at nucleotide position 1201 in exon 2 of the hGR gene, resulting in aspartic acid (D) to histidine (H) substitution at amino acid position 401 in the NTD of the receptor. Functional studies showed that compared with the wild-type hGRα, the hGRαD401H demonstrated a 2.4-fold increase in its ability to transactivate the glucocorticoid-responsive genes

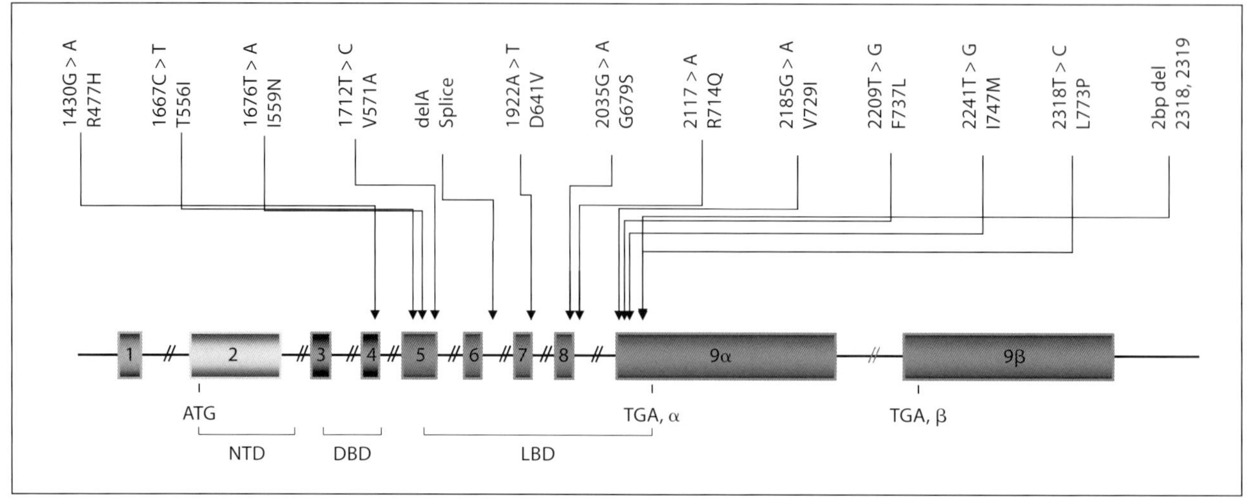

Fig. 3. Location of the known mutations of the hGR gene causing Chrousos syndrome.

and exerted a dominant positive effect upon the wild-type receptor at low concentrations. The mutant receptor hGRαD401H had similar affinity for the ligand and time to nuclear translocation, it preserved its ability to bind to GREs, and displayed a normal interaction with the GRIP1 coactivator [28] (table 2).

The impact of the mutation on the structure of the LBD of the hGRα has been examined only for hGRαR714Q. Structural changes of the mutant receptors may underlie the functional defects observed in the above-indicated functional assay systems, such as those for affinity to the ligand (ligand-binding pocket) and interaction with the GRIP1 LXXLL coactivator motif (AF2 transactivation surface). Previously reported crystallographic analyses on the hGRα LBD revealed that it consists of 12 α-helices and 4 β-sheets, which fold into a three-layer structure [42]. In the 3-D crystallographic structural model of the wild-type hGRα LBD bound to dexamethasone, arginine (R) 714 is located in the C-terminal portion of the helix 10, and a large positively charged side chain of this amino acid protrudes into a space created by helices 7, 8, 9 and 10, where this residue forms a salt bridge with glutamic acid (E) 662 located in helix 8 [23] (fig. 4a). In hGRαR714Q LBD, the arginine (R) residue is replaced by glutamine (Q), which has a smaller, uncharged side chain; thus, the mutation breaks the salt bridge with E662, and instead forms a stable new salt bridge with arginine (R) 704 of helix 9 (fig. 4b). This change in electrostatic bonding displaces helix 10 from its former salt bridge constraint, leading to further conformational changes in the ligand-binding pocket (fig. 4c, d). The mutation also destabilizes the AF-2 surface and obstructs optimal binding of the LXXLL coactivator motif to this transactivation domain (fig. 4e, f). Since the arginine (R) residue at amino acid position 714 in the hGRα is preserved in the GRs of different species and in the other human nuclear receptors [23], R714 appears to play an important role in the formation of the 3-D structure of many of the nuclear receptors, including the GR.

hGR Polymorphisms

Further to the hGR gene mutations, interindividual variations in tissue sensitivity to glucocorticoids have been described within the normal population, and have been partly attributed to polymorphisms in the hGR gene. Several polymorphisms of the hGR gene have been reported to date [43–45].

The first polymorphism, ER22/23EK, consists of two linked, single-nucleotide mutations in codons 22 and 23 in exon 2 of the hGR gene (rs 6189 and rs 6190). The first nucleotide replacement in codon 22 is silent, not resulting in an amino acid change [GAG to GAA, both coding for glutamic acid (E)], but the second replacement in codon 23 (AGG to AAG) results in arginine (R) to lysine (K) substitution [45, 46]. The ER22/23EK polymorphism results in a small reduction of the transcriptional activation of glucocorticoid-responsive genes compared with the wild-type receptor, but it does not influence transcriptional repression [46]. This polymorphism reduces sensitivity to glucocorticoids, as evidenced by the higher serum cortisol concentrations and the smaller decrease in cortisol concentrations following dexamethasone suppression testing in carriers compared with non-carriers [47], and results in a phenotype that is characterized by a more favorable metabolic profile, leading to longevity. Carriers of the ER22/23EK polymorphism display relative glucocorticoid resistance, lower fasting insulin concentrations and improved insulin sensitivity, lower total and LDL cholesterol concentrations and lower C-reactive protein concentrations [45, 48]. In line with this favorable metabolic profile, the ER22/23EK polymorphism demonstrates significantly higher incidence in the oldest half of the population. At young age, a sexually dimorphic pattern in body composition has been documented in this polymorphism [49]. Finally, at an older age, carriers of the ER22/23EK polymorphism have lower risk of dementia and fewer white matter lesions in the brain compared to non-carriers [45]. The molecular mechanisms through which the ER22/23EK polymorphism produces the above effects are likely to involve a higher expression of the hGRα-A (94-kDa) isoform at the expense of the hGRα-B (91-kDa) one. Given that the latter isoform has greater transactivational activity, the shift in hGRα-A to hGRα-B expression ratio leads to an overall decrease in transcriptional activity [50] (fig. 5).

Further downstream in exon 2, a polymorphism was identified that changes codon 363 from AAT to AGT (rs 6195), resulting in a serine (N) for asparagine (S) substitution. The N363S polymorphism is associated with higher sensitivity to glucocorticoids in vivo, resulting in an increase in the transcriptional activation of glucocorticoid-responsive genes compared with the wild-type receptor, although it does not influence transcriptional repression [46]. The N363S polymorphism is associated with higher sensitivity to glucocorticoids in vivo, increased insulin response to exogenous dexamethasone administration [45, 51], higher body mass index, higher

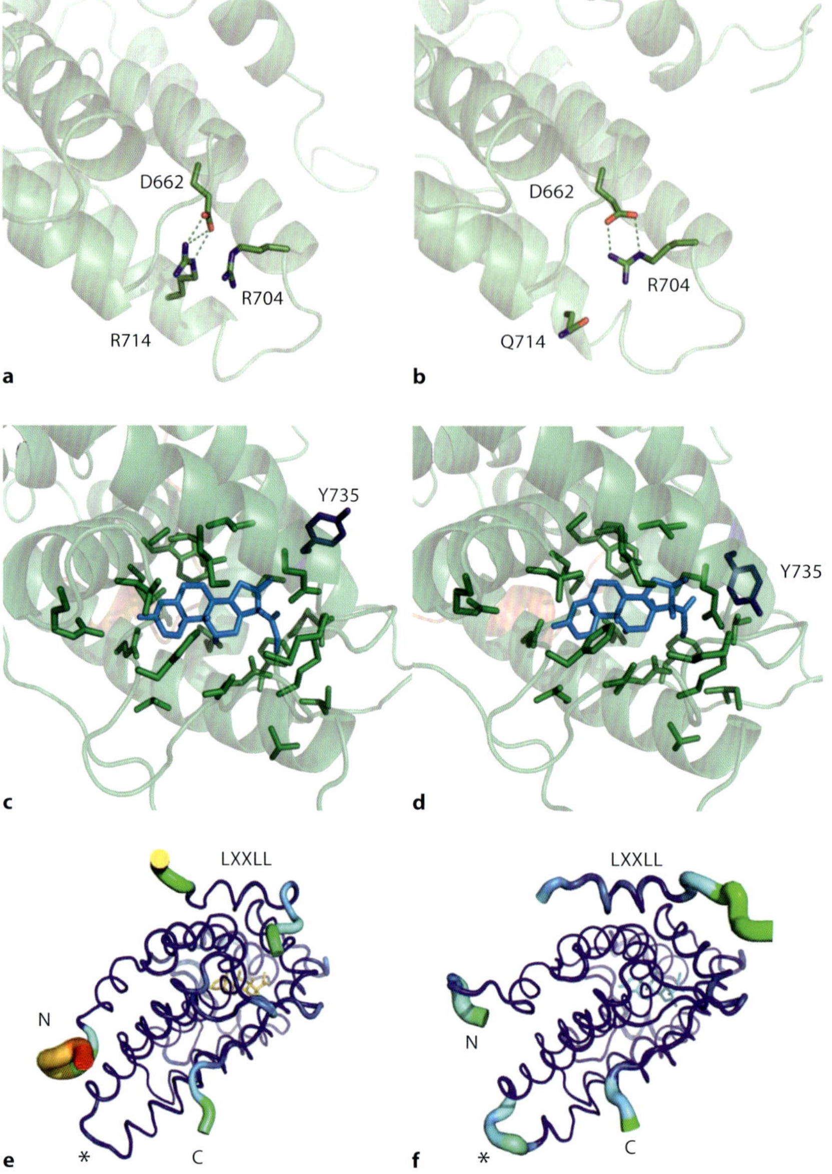

Fig. 4. Arginine (R) to glutamine (Q) replacement at amino acid 714 of the hGRα alters 3-D structure of its LBD. **a**, **b** Arginine (R) to glutamine (Q) replacement at amino acid 714 of the hGRα causes formation of a new salt bridge between arginine (R) at 704 and aspartic acid (D) at 662. **a** In the wild-type hGRα LBD, R714 is tightly bound to D662 through an electrostatic salt bridge. **b** Substitution of arginine by glutamine in the hGRαR714Q LBD results in a rearrangement of the side chains, forming a new salt bridge between R704 and D662, while displacing Q714. This relaxes some constraint on helix 10 and results in structural changes throughout the LBD. **c**, **d** hGRαR714Q LBD has altered ligand-binding pocket. The ligand-binding pocket of the wild-type hGRα (**c**) and hGRαR714Q (**d**) are shown. Arginine to glutamine replacement at amino acid 714 causes alteration in the ligand-binding pocket in hGRαR714Q LBD. The greatest change observed between the wild-type hGRα LBD and hGRαR714Q LBD is in the rotameric state of Y735. **e**, **f** hGRαR714Q LBD has the destabilized AF-2 surface that blocks optimal binding of the LXXLL coactivator motif. The thickness and color of the Cα trace of the wild-type hGRα

waist-to-hip ratio, a tendency toward lower bone mineral density in trabecular bone, elevated cholesterol and triglyceride concentrations, and higher incidence of coronary artery disease independent of weight [45, 51–57] (fig. 5).

A frequent *BclI* restriction fragment length polymorphism (rs 41423247) is also associated with increased sensitivity to glucocorticoids, hypertension, visceral adiposity [45, 58, 59] and increased insulin concentrations in obese women [60]. The exact mutation of this polymorphic site was identified as a C→G substitution in intron 2. In the elderly, the G allele of the *BclI* polymorphism is associated with a tendency towards lower lean body mass, which is likely to arise as a result of the increased sensitivity to glucocorticoids [61] (fig. 5).

The *TthIIII* variant (rs10052957) is a restriction site length polymorphism in the promoter region of the hGR gene, which is not functional by itself [45]. However, the ER22/23EK variant was invariably linked to the *TthIIII* polymorphism. Therefore, associations with glucocorticoid resistance and healthier metabolic profile observed in the *TthIIII* carriers are likely to arise as a result of the ER22/23EK polymorphism.

Finally, a single-nucleotide polymorphism that replaces A with G at the nucleoside 3669 (A3669G; rs 6198) located in the 3′ end of exon 9β has also been described [62]. This polymorphism does not change the amino acid sequence, but increases the stability of hGRβ mRNA and hGRβ protein expression, leading to greater inhibition of hGRα-induced transcriptional activity and glucocorticoid resistance. The presence of the A3669G allele is associated with reduced central obesity and a more favorable lipid profile in affected subjects [62]. Furthermore, this polymorphism selectively affects the transrepressive activity of the GR and is associated with an increased inflammatory state, rheumatoid arthritis and cardiovascular disease [63–68].

Clinical Evaluation

The first step in evaluating a patient with suspected alterations in tissue sensitivity to glucocorticoids is to obtain a complete personal and family history, with particular attention to evidence suggesting alterations in the activity of the HPA axis. In female subjects, the regularity of menstrual cycles should be documented. In children and adolescents, growth and sexual maturation should be evaluated carefully. The physical examination should include an assessment for signs of hyperandrogenism, virilization and glucocorticoid excess. Arterial blood pressure should be recorded and preferably monitored over a 24-hour period.

LBD (**e**) and hGRαR714Q LBD (**f**) indicate the areas of least (thin and blue) to most (thick and red) motion over the course of the simulation. As expected, the termini of the LBD and the bound peptide move the most. **f** There is significant motion at the mutation site (asterisk) in the mutant LBD, but not in the wild-type LBD, suggesting that the mutation causes destabilization in this structural area. The bound LXXLL peptide is, thus, more labile in the mutant LBD structure, as seen by the thickness of its Cα trace.

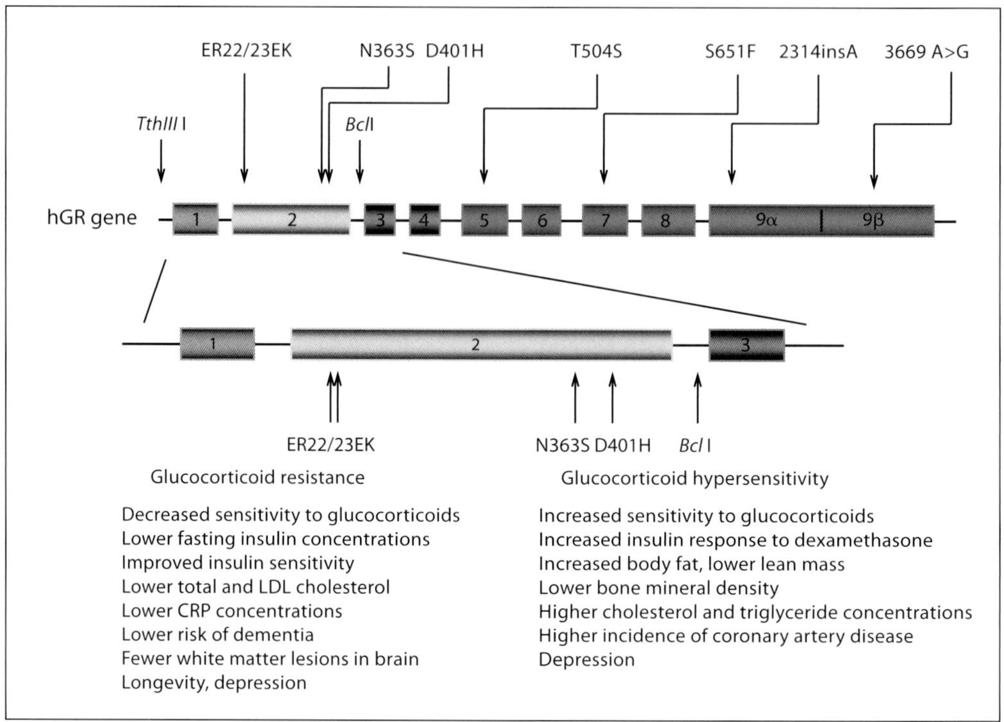

Fig. 5. Schematic representation of the hGR gene polymorphisms located in the amino-terminal domain of the receptor and a summary of their clinical associations. CRP = C-reactive protein.

Endocrinologic Evaluation

The concentrations of plasma ACTH, plasma renin activity (recumbent and upright) and aldosterone, as well as those of serum cortisol, testosterone, androstenedione, DHEA, DHEAS, total cholesterol, HDL, LDL, triglycerides, and fasting glucose and insulin should be recorded in the morning. Determination of the 24-hour (h) urinary free cortisol (UFC) excretion on 2 or 3 consecutive days is central to the diagnosis, given that patients with Chrousos syndrome demonstrate increased 24-hour UFC excretion in the absence of clinical manifestations suggestive of hypercortisolism. In patients with Chrousos syndrome, the rise in serum cortisol and androgen concentrations, as well as in the 24-hour UFC excretion varies considerably depending on the severity of impairment of glucocorticoid signal transduction. In most severe cases, serum cortisol and 24-hour UFC concentrations may be, respectively, up to 7-fold higher and 50-fold higher than the upper limit of normal range. Plasma ACTH concentrations may be normal or high in Chrousos syndrome and normal or low in PGGH.

The responsiveness of the HPA axis to exogenous glucocorticoids should also be tested with dexamethasone in patients suspected to have Chrousos syndrome. Increasing doses of dexamethasone should be given orally at midnight every other day, and a serum sample should be drawn at 08:00 h the following morning for determination of serum cortisol and dexamethasone concentrations. The concurrent measurement of serum dexamethasone concentrations is suggested in order to exclude the possibility of nonadherence to treatment, increased metabolic clearance or decreased absorption of this medication. Affected subjects demonstrate resistance of the HPA axis to dexamethasone suppression, which varies depending on the severity of the condition.

Molecular Studies

Thymidine incorporation assays and dexamethasone-binding assays on peripheral blood mononuclear cells in association with sequencing of the hGR gene are necessary to confirm the diagnosis [28, 29–40]. In Chrousos syndrome, the thymidine incorporation assays reveal resistance to dexamethasone-induced suppression of phytohemaglutinin-stimulated thymidine incorporation, while the dexamethasone-binding assays often show decreased affinity of the hGR receptor for the ligand compared to control subjects [22, 27]. The opposite is true for patients with PGGH. Sequencing of the coding region of the hGR gene, including the intron/exon junctions, will reveal mutations or deletions in most but not all cases with Chrousos syndrome [27, 29–40].

Management

In Chrousos syndrome, the aim of treatment is to suppress the excess secretion of ACTH, thereby suppressing the increased production of adrenal steroids with mineralocorticoid and androgenic activity. Treatment involves administration of high doses of mineralocorticoid-sparing synthetic glucocorticoids, such as dexamethasone (1–3 mg given once daily), which activate the mutant and/or wild-type hGRα, and suppress the endogenous secretion of ACTH in affected subjects [20–22]. It is important to achieve adequate suppression of the HPA axis to prevent the development of an ACTH-secreting adenoma in the pituitary gland and an adrenocortical adenoma in the adrenal glands [29]. Long-term dexamethasone treatment should be carefully titrated according to the clinical manifestations and biochemical profile of the affected subjects [20–22]. In PGGH, treatment aims to address the manifestations of glucocorticoid hypersensitivity, such as dyslipidemia, diabetes type 2 and hypertension [28].

Conclusions

The GR is a ubiquitously expressed intracellular, ligand-dependent transcription factor, which mediates the action of glucocorticoids and influences physiologic functions essential for life. The stochastic nature of glucocorticoid signaling pathways in association with the variable effect that hGR gene mutations/polymorphisms might have on glucocorticoid signal transduction indicates that alterations in hGR action may have important implications for many critical biological processes, such as the behavioral and physiologic responses to stress, the immune and inflammatory reaction, the process of sleep, as well as basic functions, such as growth and reproduction. In clinical practice, the effects of glucocorticoid treatment may vary considerably between patients, and may be partly attributed to mutations or polymorphisms in the hGR gene. Therefore, when the presence of these hGR gene variants is known, the dose of glucocorticoids should be adjusted accordingly to ensure optimal therapy and minimal adverse effects.

References

1 Kino T, Chrousos GP: Glucocorticoid effects on gene expression; in Steckler T, Kalin NH, Reul JMHM (eds): Handbook of Stress and the Brain. Amsterdam, Elsevier, 2005, pp 295–311.

2 Chrousos GP, Charmandari E, Kino T: Glucocorticoid action networks – an introduction to systems biology. J Clin Endocrinol Metab 2004;89:563–564.

3 Chrousos GP: The glucocorticoid receptor gene, longevity, and the complex disorders of Western societies. Am J Med 2004;117;204–207.

4 Galon J, Franchimont D, Hiroi N, Frey G, Boettner A, Ehrhart-Bornstein M, O'Shea JJ, Chrousos GP, Bornstein SR: Gene profiling reveals unknown enhancing and suppressive actions of glucocorticoids on immune cells. FASEB J 2002;16:61–71.

5 Zhou J, Cidlowski JA: The human glucocorticoid receptor: one gene, multiple proteins and diverse responses. Steroids 2005;70:407–417.

6 Duma D, Jewell CM, Cidlowski JA: Multiple glucocorticoid receptor isoforms and mechanisms of post-translational modification. J Steroid Biochem Mol Biol 2006;102:11–21.

7 Nicolaides NC, Galata Z, Kino T, Chrousos GP, Charmandari E: The human glucocorticoid receptor: molecular basis of biologic function. Steroids 2010;75:1–12.

8 Hollenberg SM, Weinberger C, Ong ES, Cerelli G, Oro A, Lebo R, Thompson EB, Rosenfeld MG, Evans RM: Primary structure and expression of a functional human glucocorticoid receptor cDNA. Nature 1985;318:635–641.

9 Kino T, Manoli I, Kelkar S, Wang Y, Su YA, Chrousos GP: Glucocorticoid receptor (GR) β has intrinsic, GRα-independent transcriptional activity. Biochem Biophys Res Commun 2009;381:671–675.

10 Oakley RH, Jewell CM, Yudt MR, Bofetiado DM, Cidlowski JA: The dominant negative activity of the human glucocorticoid receptor β isoform. Specificity and mechanisms of action. J Biol Chem 1999; 274:27857–27866.

11 Chrousos GP, Kino T: Intracellular glucocorticoid signaling: a formerly simple system turns stochastic. Sci STKE 2005;2005:pe48.

12 McKenna NJ, Lanz RB, O'Malley BW: Nuclear receptor coregulators: cellular and molecular biology. Endocr Rev 1999;20:321–344.

13 McKenna NJ, O'Malley BW: Combinatorial control of gene expression by nuclear receptors and coregulators. Cell 2002;108:465–474.

14 Auboeuf D, Honig A, Berget SM, O'Malley BW: Coordinate regulation of transcription and splicing by steroid receptor coregulators. Science 2002;298: 416–419.

15 Hittelman AB, Burakov D, Iniguez-Lluhi JA, Freedman LP, Garabedian MJ: Differential regulation of glucocorticoid receptor transcriptional activation via AF-1-associated proteins. EMBO J 1999;18: 5380–5388.

16 Liu J, DeFranco DB: Protracted nuclear export of glucocorticoid receptor limits its turnover and does not require the exportin 1/CRM1-directed nuclear export pathway. Mol Endocrinol 2000;14:40–51.

17 Chrousos GP: Hormone resistance and hypersensitivity states; in Chrousos GP, Olefsky JM, Samols E (eds): Modern Endocrinology Series. Philadelphia, Lippincott, Williams & Wilkins, 2002, p 542.
18 Kino T, De Martino MU, Charmandari E, Mirani M, Chrousos GP: Tissue glucocorticoid resistance/hypersensitivity syndromes. J Steroid Biochem Mol Biol 2003;85:457–467.
19 Chrousos GP, Kino T: Glucocorticoid signaling in the cell. Expanding clinical implications to complex human behavioral and somatic disorders. Proc NY Acad Sci 2009;1179:153–166.
20 Chrousos GP, Vingerhoeds A, Brandon D, Eil C, Pugeat M, DeVroede M, Loriaux DL, Lipsett MB: Primary cortisol resistance in man. A glucocorticoid receptor-mediated disease. J Clin Invest 1982; 69:1261–1269.
21 Chrousos GP, Detera-Wadleigh SD, Karl M: Syndromes of glucocorticoid resistance. Ann Intern Med 1993;119:1113–1124.
22 Charmandari E, Kino T, Ichijo T, Chrousos GP: Generalized glucocorticoid resistance: clinical aspects, molecular mechanisms, and implications of a rare genetic disorder. J Clin Endocrinol Metab 2008;93:1563–1572.
23 Nader N, Bachrach BE, Hurt DE, Gajula S, Pittman A, Lescher R, Kino T: A novel point mutation in the helix 10 of the human glucocorticoid receptor causes generalized glucocorticoid resistance by disrupting the structure of the ligand-binding domain. J Clin Endocrinol Metab 2010;95:2281–2285.
24 McMahon SK, Pretorius CJ, Ungerer JP, Salmon NJ, Conwell LS, Pearen MA, Batch JA: Neonatal complete generalized glucocorticoid resistance and growth hormone deficiency caused by a novel homozygous mutation in Helix 12 of the ligand binding domain of the glucocorticoid receptor gene (NR3C1). J Clin Endocrinol Metab 2010;95:297–302.
25 Tomlinson JW, Walker EA, Bujalska IJ, Draper N, Lavery GG, Cooper MS, Hewison M, Stewart PM: 11β-hydroxysteroid dehydrogenase type 1: a tissue-specific regulator of glucocorticoid response. Endocr Rev 2004;25:831–866.
26 Charmandari E, Kino T: Chrousos syndrome: a seminal report, a phylogenetic enigma and the clinical implications of glucocorticoid signalling changes. Eur J Clin Invest 2010;40:932–942.
27 Chrousos G: Q&A: primary generalized glucocorticoid resistance. BMC Med 2011;9:27.
28 Charmandari E, Ichijo T, Jubiz W, Baid S, Zachman K, Chrousos GP, Kino T: A novel point mutation in the amino terminal domain of the human glucocorticoid receptor (hGR) gene enhancing hGR-mediated gene expression. J Clin Endocrinol Metab 2008;93:4963–4968.
29 Karl M, Lamberts SW, Koper JW, Katz DA, Huizenga NE, Kino T, Haddad BR, Hughes MR, Chrousos GP: Cushing's disease preceded by generalized glucocorticoid resistance: clinical consequences of a novel, dominant-negative glucocorticoid receptor mutation. Proc Assoc Am Physicians 1996;108: 296–307.
30 Hurley DM, Accili D, Stratakis CA, Karl M, Vamvakopoulos N, Rorer E, Constantine K, Taylor SI, Chrousos GP: Point mutation causing a single amino acid substitution in the hormone binding domain of the glucocorticoid receptor in familial glucocorticoid resistance. J Clin Invest 1991;87: 680–686.
31 Karl M, Lamberts SW, Detera-Wadleigh SD, Encio IJ, Stratakis CA, Hurley DM, Accili D, Chrousos GP: Familial glucocorticoid resistance caused by a splice site deletion in the human glucocorticoid receptor gene. J Clin Endocrinol Metab 1993;76: 683–689.
32 Malchoff DM, Brufsky A, Reardon G, McDermott P, Javier EC, Bergh CH, Rowe D, Malchoff CD: A mutation of the glucocorticoid receptor in primary cortisol resistance. J Clin Invest 1993;91:1918–1925.
33 Kino T, Stauber RH, Resau JH, Pavlakis GN, Chrousos GP: Pathologic human GR mutant has a transdominant negative effect on the wild-type GR by inhibiting its translocation into the nucleus: importance of the ligand-binding domain for intracellular GR trafficking. J Clin Endocrinol Metab 2001;86: 5600–5608.
34 Ruiz M, Lind U, Gafvels M, Eggertsen G, Carlstedt-Duke J, Nilsson L, Holtmann M, Stierna P, Wikstrom AC, Werner S: Characterization of two novel mutations in the glucocorticoid receptor gene in patients with primary cortisol resistance. Clin Endocrinol (Oxf) 2001;55:363–371.
35 Mendonca BB, Leite MV, de Castro M, Kino T, Elias LL, Bachega TA, Arnhold IJ, Chrousos GP, Latronico AC: Female pseudohermaphroditism caused by a novel homozygous missense mutation of the GR gene. J Clin Endocrinol Metab 2002;87:1805–1809.
36 Vottero A, Kino T, Combe H, Lecomte P, Chrousos GP: A novel, C-terminal dominant negative mutation of the GR causes familial glucocorticoid resistance through abnormal interactions with p160 steroid receptor coactivators. J Clin Endocrinol Metab 2002;87:2658–2667.
37 Charmandari E, Kino T, Vottero A, Souvatzoglou E, Bhattacharyya N, Chrousos GP: Natural glucocorticoid receptor mutants causing generalized glucocorticoid resistance: molecular genotype, genetic transmission and clinical phenotype. J Clin Endocrinol Metab 2004;89:1939–1949.

38 Charmandari E, Raji A, Kino T, Ichijo T, Tiulpakov A, Zachman K, Chrousos GP: A novel point mutation in the ligand-binding domain (LBD) of the human glucocorticoid receptor (hGR) causing generalized glucocorticoid resistance: the importance of the C terminus of hGR LBD in conferring transactivational activity. J Clin Endocrinol Metab 2005; 90:3696–3705.

39 Charmandari E, Kino T, Ichijo T, Zachman K, Alatsatianos A, Chrousos GP: Functional characterization of the natural human glucocorticoid receptor (hGR) mutants hGRαR477H and hGRαG679S associated with generalized glucocorticoid resistance. J Clin Endocrinol Metab 2006;91:1535–1543.

40 Charmandari E, Kino T, Ichijo T, Jubiz W, Mejia L, Zachman K, Chrousos GP: A novel point mutation in helix 11 of the ligand-binding domain of the human glucocorticoid receptor gene causing generalized glucocorticoid resistance. J Clin Endocrinol Metab 2007;92:3986–3990.

41 Zhu HJ, Dai YF, Wang O, Li M, Lu L, Zhao WG, Xing XP, Pan H, Li NS, Gong FY: Generalized glucocorticoid resistance accompanied with an adrenocortical adenoma and caused by a novel point mutation of human glucocorticoid receptor gene. Chin Med J (Engl) 2011;124:551–555.

42 Bledsoe RK, Montana VG, Stanley TB, Delves CJ, Apolito CJ, McKee DD, Consler TG, Parks DJ, Stewart EL, Willson TM, Lambert MH, Moore JT, Pearce KH, Xu HE: Crystal structure of the glucocorticoid receptor ligand binding domain reveals a novel mode of receptor dimerization and coactivator recognition. Cell 2002;110:93–105.

43 Lamberts SW, Huizenga AT, de Lange P, de Jong FH, Koper JW: Clinical aspects of glucocorticoid sensitivity. Steroids 1996;61:157–160.

44 Smit P, Russcher H, de Jong FH, Brinkmann AO, Lamberts SW, Koper JW: Differential regulation of synthetic glucocorticoids on gene expression levels of glucocorticoid-induced leucine zipper and interleukin-2. J Clin Endocrinol Metab 2005;90: 2994–3000.

45 van Rossum EF, Lamberts SW: Polymorphisms in the glucocorticoid receptor gene and their associations with metabolic parameters and body composition. Recent Prog Horm Res 2004;59:333–357.

46 Russcher H, Smit P, van den Akker EL, van Rossum EF, Brinkmann AO, de Jong FH, Lamberts SW, Koper JW: Two polymorphisms in the glucocorticoid receptor gene directly affect glucocorticoid-regulated gene expression. J Clin Endocrinol Metab 2005;90:5804–5810.

47 van Rossum EF, Koper JW, Huizenga NA, Uitterlinden AG, Janssen JA, Brinkmann AO, Grobbee DE, de Jong FH, van Duyn CM, Pols HA, Lamberts SW: A polymorphism in the glucocorticoid receptor gene, which decreases sensitivity to glucocorticoids in vivo, is associated with low insulin and cholesterol levels. Diabetes 2002;51:3128–3134.

48 van Rossum EF, Feelders RA, van den Beld AW, Uitterlinden AG, Janssen JA, Ester W, Brinkmann AO, Grobbee DE, de Jong FH, Pols HA, Koper JW, Lamberts SW: Association of the ER22/23EK polymorphism in the glucocorticoid receptor gene with survival and C-reactive protein levels in elderly men. Am J Med 2004;117:158–162.

49 van Rossum EF, Voorhoeve PG, te Velde SJ, Koper JW, Delemarre-van de Waal HA, Kemper HC, Lamberts SW: The ER22/23EK polymorphism in the glucocorticoid receptor gene is associated with a beneficial body composition and muscle strength in young adults. J Clin Endocrinol Metab 2004;89: 4004–4009.

50 Russcher H, van Rossum EF, de Jong FH, Brinkmann AO, Lamberts SW, Koper JW: Increased expression of the glucocorticoid receptor-A translational isoform as a result of the ER22/23EK polymorphism. Mol Endocrinol 2005;19:1687–1696.

51 Huizenga NA, Koper JW, De Lange P, Pols HA, Stolk RP, Burger H, Grobbee DE, Brinkmann AO, De Jong FH, Lamberts SW: A polymorphism in the glucocorticoid receptor gene may be associated with and increased sensitivity to glucocorticoids in vivo. J Clin Endocrinol Metab 1998;83:144–151.

52 Lin RC, Wang XL, Dalziel B, Caterson ID, Morris BJ: Association of obesity, but not diabetes or hypertension, with glucocorticoid receptor N363S variant. Obes Res 2003;11:802–808.

53 Di Blasio AM, van Rossum EF, Maestrini S, Berselli ME, Tagliaferri M, Podestà F, Koper JW, Liuzzi A, Lamberts SW: The relation between two polymorphisms in the glucocorticoid receptor gene and body mass index, blood pressure and cholesterol in obese patients. Clin Endocrinol (Oxf) 2003;59: 68–74.

54 Roussel R, Reis AF, Dubois-Laforgue D, Bellanné-Chantelot C, Timsit J, Velho G: The N363S polymorphism in the glucocorticoid receptor gene is associated with overweight in subjects with type 2 diabetes mellitus. Clin Endocrinol (Oxf) 2003;59: 237–241.

55 Dobson MG, Redfern CP, Unwin N, Weaver JU: The N363S polymorphism of the glucocorticoid receptor: potential contribution to central obesity in men and lack of association with other risk factors for coronary heart disease and diabetes mellitus. J Clin Endocrinol Metab 2001;86:2270–2274.

56 Lin RC, Wang XL, Morris BJ: Association of coronary artery disease with glucocorticoid receptor N363S variant. Hypertension 2003;41:404–407.
57 Szabó V, Borgulya G, Filkorn T, Majnik J, Bányász I, Nagy ZZ: The variant N363S of glucocorticoid receptor in steroid-induced ocular hypertension in Hungarian patients treated with photorefractive keratectomy. Mol Vis 2007;13:659–666.
58 Rosmond R, Chagnon YC, Holm G, Chagnon M, Pérusse L, Lindell K, Carlsson B, Bouchard C, Björntorp P: A glucocorticoid receptor gene marker is associated with abdominal obesity, leptin, and dysregulation of the hypothalamic-pituitary-adrenal axis. Obes Res 2000;8:211–218.
59 Ukkola O, Pérusse L, Chagnon YC, Després JP, Bouchard C: Interactions among the glucocorticoid receptor, lipoprotein lipase and adrenergic receptor genes and abdominal fat in the Québec Family Study. Int J Obes Relat Metab Disord 2001;25: 1332–1339.
60 Weaver JU, Hitman GA, Kopelman PG: An association between a BclI restriction fragment length polymorphism of the glucocorticoid receptor locus and hyperinsulinaemia in obese women. J Mol Endocrinol 1992;9:295–300.
61 van Rossum EF, Koper JW, van den Beld AW, Uitterlinden AG, Arp P, Ester W, Janssen JA, Brinkmann AO, de Jong FH, Grobbee DE, Pols HA, Lamberts SW: Identification of the BclI polymorphism in the glucocorticoid receptor gene: association with sensitivity to glucocorticoids in vivo and body mass index. Clin Endocrinol (Oxf) 2003;59: 585–592.
62 Syed AA, Irving JA, Redfern CP, Hall AG, Unwin NC, White M, Bhopal RS, Weaver JU: Association of glucocorticoid receptor polymorphism A3669G in exon 9beta with reduced central adiposity in women. Obesity (Silver Spring) 2006;14:759–764.
63 Lee EB, Kim JY, Lee YJ, Song YW: Glucocorticoid receptor polymorphisms in Korean patients with rheumatoid arthritis. Ann Rheum Dis 2005;64: 503–504.
64 van den Akker EL, Russcher H, van Rossum EF, Brinkmann AO, de Jong FH, Hokken A, Pols HA, Koper JW, Lamberts SW: Glucocorticoid receptor polymorphism affects transrepression but not transactivation. J Clin Endocrinol Metab 2006;91: 2800–2803.
65 van den Akker EL, Nouwen JL, Melles DC, van Rossum EF, Koper JW, Uitterlinden AG, Hofman A, Verbrugh HA, Pols HA, Lamberts SW, van Belkum A: *Staphylococcus aureus* nasal carriage is associated with glucocorticoid receptor gene polymorphisms. J Infect Dis 2006;194:814–818.
66 van den Akker EL, Koper JW, van Rossum EF, Dekker MJ, Russcher H, de Jong FH, Uitterlinden AG, Hofman A, Pols HA, Witteman JC, Lamberts SW: Glucocorticoid receptor gene and risk of cardiovascular disease. Arch Intern Med 2008;168: 33–39.
67 Otte C, Wüst S, Zhao S, Pawlikowska L, Kwok PY, Whooley MA: Glucocorticoid receptor gene, low-grade inflammation, and heart failure: the Heart and Soul study. J Clin Endocrinol Metab 2010;95: 2885–2891.
68 Geelhoed JJ, van Duijn C, van Osch-Gevers L, Steegers EA, Hofman A, Helbing WA, Jaddoe VW: Glucocorticoid receptor-9beta polymorphism is associated with systolic blood pressure and heart growth during early childhood. The Generation R Study. Early Hum Dev 2011;87:97–102.

Evangelia Charmandari, MD, PhD
Division of Endocrinology and Metabolism, Clinical Research Center
Biomedical Research Foundation of the Academy of Athens
4 Soranou tou Efessiou Street, GR–11527 Athens (Greece)
E-Mail evangelia.charmandari@googlemail.com

Maghnie M, Loche S, Cappa M, Ghizzoni L, Lorini R (eds): Hormone Resistance and Hypersensitivity. From Genetics to Clinical Management. Endocr Dev. Basel, Karger, 2013, vol 24, pp 86–95 (DOI: 10.1159/000342508)

Pseudohypoaldosteronism

Felix G. Riepe

Division of Pediatric Endocrinology, Department of Pediatrics, University Hospital Schleswig-Holstein, Kiel, Germany

Abstract

Pseudohypoaldosteronism (PHA) is a rare syndrome of mineralocorticoid resistance. PHA type 1 (PHA1) can be divided into two different forms, showing either a systemic or a renal form of mineralocorticoid resistance. The first is caused by mutations of the genes coding the epithelial sodium channel, the latter is caused by mutations in the mineralocorticoid receptor coding gene *NR3C2*. The clinical manifestation of systemic PHA1 is overt dehydration and hyponatremia due to systemic salt loss and severe hyperkalemia. The leading clinical sign of the less severe renal PHA1 is insufficient weight gain due to chronic dehydration. Hyperkalemia is generally mild. The patients manifest clinical signs mainly in early infancy. In both entities, plasma renin and aldosterone concentrations are highly elevated, reflecting a resistance of the kidney and other tissues to mineralocorticoids. PHA2 is characterized by hyperkalemia and hypertension. It has been described by Gordon's group as a syndrome with highly variable plasma aldosterone concentrations, suppressed plasma renin activity, various degrees of hyperchloremia and metabolic acidosis. PHA3 comprises transient and secondary forms of salt-losing states caused by various pathologies. Urinary tract infections and obstructive uropathies are the most frequent cause. Contrary to PHA1 and PHA2, the glomerular filtration rate is decreased in PHA3.

Aldosterone is the key regulator of transepithelial sodium transport. Sodium and potassium balance, blood pressure and fluid homeostasis are maintained by the effect of aldosterone on polarized epithelial cells. The mineralocorticoid receptor (MR) and the amiloride-sensitive epithelial sodium channel (ENaC) are the leading intracellular actors necessary for sodium conservation mediated by aldosterone. Dysfunction of the intracellular aldosterone signaling pathway leads to pseudohypoaldosteronism (PHA). The discovery of the underlying molecular defects in PHA gave major insights into the intracellular factors responsible for salt homeostasis and their interaction as transepithelial sodium transport machinery.

The Mineralocorticoid Receptor

The MR is a member of the classic steroid-thyroid-retinoid nuclear receptor family. These receptors act as ligand-dependent transcription factors that regulate a variety of physiological processes. The human *NR3C2* gene codes for the MR. It is localized on chromosome 4q31.1 and contains about 450 kb [1]. *NR3C2* is composed of ten exons, whereas the first two exons (1α and 1β) are untranslated. The MR protein contains 984 amino acids organized in three domains, including the N-terminal domain, the DNA-binding domain and the C-terminal ligand-binding domain (LBD). Tissue-specific translation of MR is achieved by different mRNA isoforms originating from the transcription of exon 1α and 1β, utilization of cryptic splice sites at the exon 3/intron C splice junction, exon skipping of exon 5 and/or exon 6 or the control of gene expression by two promoters with different transcriptional activity. The MR harbors potential phosphorylated residues and can be ubiquitinylated and sumoylated. All these mechanisms allow posttranslational tissue-specific modification of MR activity and specificity. As with other nuclear receptors, a ligand-dependent interaction of the N-terminal domain and the LBD was detected [2]. The DNA-binding domain is the region that defines the nuclear receptor superfamily. Two zinc fingers are formed by two groups of four cysteines which bind two zinc atoms. These zinc fingers are responsible for the sequence-specific contact to the DNA [1]. The MR LBD crystal structure has been studied [3]. It consists of eleven α-helices with four β-strands folded into a helical structure with three different layers. A loop between helix 6 and 7 was identified as the key structure regulating the hormone specificity of MR. The key residue in this loop is L848, which partially precludes C17 hydroxylated steroids such as cortisol from binding. The interaction of helix 10 and 12 is critical for MR activation. The conformational change of the position of helix 12 with ligand binding facilitates the binding of coactivator molecules. The interaction with coactivators and corepressors significantly modifies the MR activation. However, no salt-losing phenotype was detected in knockouts for steroid receptor coactivators.

The Epithelial Sodium Channel

ENaC constitutes the rate-limiting step in sodium reabsorption in the apical membrane of epithelia [4]. It is characterized by a high selectivity for sodium and a high affinity for the potassium-sparing diuretics amiloride and triamterene. ENaC is a heteromultimeric protein consisting of three subunits, termed α-, β- and γ-ENaC. The α-, β- and γ-ENaC subunits are coded by the *SCNN1A* gene on chromosome 12p13, and the *SCNN1B* and the *SCNN1G* genes on chromosome 16p12. As deduced from the crystal structure of the ENaC orthologue ASIC1 channel, ENaC is likely a trimer consisting of three homologous subunits α, β and γ [5]. All three subunits share about

35% homology at the amino acid level and adopt the same topology, with two transmembrane α-helices, a short intracellular amino- and carboxy-terminal end and a large extracellular loop corresponding to about two thirds of the protein. Numerous lysine residues in the amino-terminal region can be ubiquitinated, and are key elements determining the half-life of the channel [6]. The extracellular loop contains several glycosylation sites as well as two cysteine-rich boxes which are critical for channel trafficking to the cell membrane. The intracellular carboxy-terminus contains several functional domains involved in the regulation of the number of channels present at the cell surface. A proline-rich domain in the carboxy-terminus resembles an SH3 protein-protein interaction domain, and is involved in the interaction with the cytoskeleton.

Sodium Reabsorption at Tight Epithelia

In the kidney, aldosterone mainly acts in the collecting duct regulating the final urinary sodium and potassium concentration [7]. Filtrated sodium is reabsorbed from the glomerular filtrate through a tight epithelium formed by principal and intercalated cells. Tight junctions are responsible for the intercellular sealing of these cells. The aldosterone-mediated sodium reabsorption utilizes a transepithelial transport machinery consisting of various intracytoplasmatic, nuclear and transmembranous proteins (fig. 1). This facilitated transport of sodium through tight epithelia is comparable in the distal tubule of the kidney, the colon and the salivary and sweat glands. Sodium crosses the apical epithelial membrane electrogenically through the ion-selective ENaC. The active transport at the basolateral membrane is mediated by the Na, K-ATPase [8]. This generates a lumen-negative voltage that drives K^+ secretion facilitated through a selective potassium channel (ROMK) into the lumen. Both cations are transported against an electrochemical potential with large transtubular concentration gradients of up to 1:3 for Na^+, and 20:1 for K^+ (lumen:interstitial fluid). Aldosterone regulates these channels by binding to its intracellular MR after passively crossing the epithelial membrane. The ligand-bound receptor translocates into the nucleus and concentrates in prominent intranuclear clusters in the case of bound MR agonists, whereas no cluster formation occurs with MR antagonists. The MR has a comparable affinity to mineralocorticoids and glucocorticoids. Without regulation at a prereceptor level, the MR would be fully occupied by cortisol because its concentration is at least an order of magnitude greater than that of aldosterone. The coexpression of the enzyme 11β-hydroxysteroid dehydrogenase type 2 in epithelial cells safeguards the MR from cortisol occupation via metabolization of cortisol to cortisone, which has no affinity to the receptor. Ligand-bound MR binds as a dimer to response elements in the promoter regions of aldosterone target genes and initiates hormone-mediated gene transcription or repression. The genomic action of aldosterone can be divided into an early and a late phase. The existing

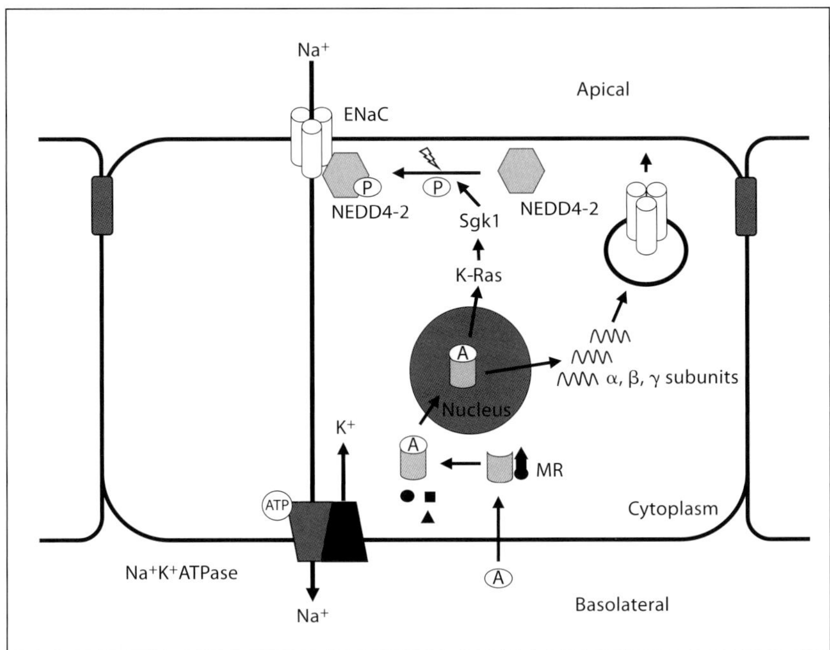

Fig. 1. Schematic illustration of the transepithelial sodium reabsorption machinery. Aldosterone binds to the intracytoplasmatic MR after the dissociation of chaperone proteins such as heat shock protein. The aldosterone-MR complex translocates into the nucleus and binds to specific DNA sequences and induces or represses the transcription of different hormone-responsive genes. Among others, these genes include signaling factors like K-Ras which can activate SGK1. SGK1 phosphorylates NEDD4-2 and others facilitating the interaction with ENaC, hereby accumulating at the plasma membrane. Through these factors, the transepithelial sodium transport is enhanced without a numerical increase in transport proteins by increasing the open probability of apical ion channels and/or by increasing the number of active apical ion channels. During the late phase of aldosterone action, the transcription and translation of ENaC subunits, Na^+K^+ATPase and other factors of the sodium transport machinery are enhanced (see text for details).

transport machinery is activated by the transcription of signaling factors during the early phase. Well-studied early induced signaling factors are *SGK1* [9] and genes of the Ras familiy, such as *K-Ras* [10]. Through these factors, the transepithelial sodium transport is enhanced without a numerical increase in transport proteins. As the capacity of the basolateral Na^+/K^+ATPase is not considered to be limiting during the early phase of aldosterone action, the signaling factors can enhance the aldosterone-mediated sodium transport by increasing the open probability of apical ion channels and/or by increasing the number of active apical ion channels. Serum- and glucocorticoid-induced kinase 1 (Sgk1) is believed to increase the number of ENaC in the apical membrane. Sgk1 is an inducible Ser/Thr kinase. After protein translation, Sgk1 is activated by phosphorylation [11]. Activated Sgk1 phosphorylates Nedd4-2 (neuronal precursor cell expressed developmentally downregulated

2) which allows binding of 14-3-3 proteins [12]. This alleviates the Nedd4-2/ENaC interaction, causing a reduced ubiquitylation and hereby an accumulation of epithelial sodium channels (ENaC) at the plasma membrane. K-Ras can activate phosphatidyl inositol 3-kinase which can activate 3-phosphoinositide-dependent protein kinase 1 whose target is Sgk1 [11]. Thus, K-Ras might control Sgk1, and both factors might be integral parts of various convergent intracellular signal cascades. During the late phase of aldosterone action, there is an increase in the amount of ENaC protein in the cell, although there is controversy regarding which subunit of the heteromultimeric ENaC is induced by aldosterone. The number of basolateral Na^+K^+ATPase also increases in response to aldosterone. The apical K^+ channel (ROMK) transcription is identically increased in response to aldosterone in order to keep up the electrogenic potential of the epithelial cell.

Pseudohypoaldosteronism

PHA is a rare heterogeneous syndrome of mineralocorticoid resistance resulting in insufficient potassium and hydrogen secretion. Therefore, the three mandatory clinical features are hyperkalemia, metabolic acidosis and elevated plasma aldosterone levels. Salt wasting is an additional feature in two subtypes of PHA. PHA has been classified into three distinct forms. This classification includes primarily salt losing syndromes, such as PHA1 and PHA3 and the potassium retaining syndrome PHA2, which are all caused by a form of mineralocorticoid resistance due to disturbances in the mineralocorticoid-mediated signal transduction machinery (table 1).

PHA Type 1

PHA type 1 (PHA1) is a rare inherited disease characterized by neonatal salt loss resistant to mineralocorticoid treatment, which was first described by Cheek and Perry in 1958 [13]. Clinical features are severe salt wasting, life-threatening hyperkalemia, metabolic acidosis, dehydration and failure to thrive. Plasma renin and aldosterone concentrations are excessively elevated, reflecting a peripheral resistance to mineralocorticoids. Adrenal function is not impaired in these patients. Only treatment with salt supplementation is effective in PHA1. In addition, ion exchange resins sometimes have to be given in order to lower the elevated potassium level. Two forms of PHA1 can be distinguished at the clinical and molecular level [14]. The severity of the disease and the phenotype of the two genetically different PHA1 forms vary strikingly.

The multi-organ sPHA1 follows an autosomal recessive trait of inheritance. sPHA1 presents in the neonatal period with hyponatremia due to multi-organ salt loss, including kidneys, colon and sweat and salivary glands. Sodium concentration in sweat,

Table 1. Phenotypes in PHA

PHA type	Alternative nomenclature	Inheritance	Characteristics	Affected genes
1	systemic PHA	recessive	– systemic salt loss, severe form – hyponatremia, hyperkalemia, metabolic acidosis, elevated renin and aldosterone	*SCNN1A, SCNN1B, SCNN1G*
	renal PHA	dominant	– renal salt loss, less severe form – hyponatremia, hyperkalemia, metabolic acidosis, elevated renin and aldosterone	*NR3C2*
2	Gordon syndrome	dominant	– hyperkalemia, hypertension, hyperchloremic acidosis, suppressed renin, normal aldosterone	*WNK1, WNK4*
3	secondary PHA	none	– secondary to nephropathies, uropathies, intestinal or other salt loss – hyponatremia, hyperkalemia, metabolic acidosis, elevated renin and aldosterone, – low glomerular filtration rate	none

which is elevated, and nasal or rectal transepithelial voltage differences, which are zero, can be used as a diagnostic tool. Hyponatremia and hyperkalemia are combined with elevated plasma renin and aldosterone concentrations. Children suffering from sPHA1 often show lower respiratory tract diseases due to reduced sodium-dependent liquid absorption [15]. The airway abnormalities manifest clinically as cough, tachypnea, fever and wheezing [15]. As sPHA1 is a systemic disease, phenotypes showing cholelithiasis, skin rashes mimicking milia rubra or dermal infections, salt loss via the meibomian glands or polyhydramnios are reported. sPHA1 manifests in the first month of life, persists into adulthood and shows no improvement over time [14]. Nearly all patients require intensive care and different therapeutic approaches to lower life-threatening hyperkalemia. In some patients, i.v. sodium supplementation and the application of albuterol or glucose/insulin are sufficient to reestablish Na/K balance. Some patients, however, additionally need ion exchange resins or even dialysis. Life-long sodium supplementation as sodium chloride and sodium bicarbonate is the essential therapy. These patients are prone lifelong to life-threatening salt losing crises combined with severe hyperkalemia and dehydration.

The systemic form of PHA1 is caused by inactivating mutations of the ENaC subunit genes *SCNN1A* (chromosome 12p13.31), *SCNN1B* (chromosome 16p12.1) and *SCNN1G* (chromosome 16p12.1). The first mutations in the subunit genes were reported by Chang et al. [16] in 5 consanguineous kindreds from the Near-East. Various mutations have since been reported in the human gene mutation database (HGMD®) at the Institute of Medical Genetics in Cardiff (www.hgmd.cf.ac.uk).

Recently, a partially inactivating mutation of the *SCNN1A* gene has been detected, causing a phenotype restricted to a renal salt loss illustrating a possible continuum from systemic to renal PHA [17].

In contrast to systemic sPHA1, rPHA1 is characterized by an isolated renal resistance to aldosterone, leading to renal salt loss, hyponatremia, hyperkalemia, metabolic acidosis, failure to thrive, elevated plasma renin and aldosterone concentrations in infancy [18]. The main clinical symptom is insufficient weight gain due to chronic dehydration. Hyperkalemia is generally mild, and metabolic acidosis is not always detectable. Patients with rPHA1 show no elevated sodium levels in sweat or saliva. A pulmonary manifestation is absent. Patients mainly manifest in early infancy between 0.5 and 6 months. Treatment consists of sodium supplementation. Potassium-binding resins are rarely needed. Interestingly, the salt treatment becomes generally unnecessary by 2–3 years of age [13]. It is not known why the patients are then able to maintain electrolyte homeostasis without further treatment. Suggestions are the chronically upregulated renin-angiotensin-aldosterone system, kidney maturation or replacement of distal sodium reabsorption by proximal parts of the tubulus. Overall, rPHA1 is a milder PHA form which is strictly restricted to the kidney.

rPHA1 is caused by inactivating mutations in the human MR gene *NR3C2* [19]. This was anticipated from the experimental treatment of rPHA1 patients with carbenoxolone, which inhibits the cortisol to cortisone-converting enzyme 11β-hydroxysteroid dehydrogenase type II, which was partially able to correct the apparent mineralocorticoid resistance [20]. Carbenoxolone elevates the intracellular cortisol concentration sufficiently to activate the wild-type MR, overcoming a functional defect in the mutant receptor. The first mutations were identified by Geller et al. [19] in the late 1990s. To date, more than 50 mutations in the human *NR3C2* gene causing rPHA1 have been described. *NR3C2* mutations are found as familial or de novo mutations in a considerable part of patients [21]. These mutations are spread throughout the gene. Mutations are found in the heterozygous state, indicating that the loss of one *NR3C2* allele is enough to develop an rPHA1 phenotype. Identical *NR3C2* gene mutations in rPHA1 lead to a very heterogeneous disease expression within one affected family. The clinical spectrum ranges from healthy unaffected patients, patients without electrolyte disturbances but elevated plasma renin and aldosterone to patients with the classical disease [21]. Geller et al. [22] studied a total of 35 family members from two families with the identical MR mutation, including 14 individuals who carried the mutation and 21 individuals who did not. In one family, only the index case was symptomatic with rPHA1, whereas in the other family the index and the siblings showed signs of rPHA1, while 5 other genotypically affected individuals in the pedigree were asymptomatic. In this setting, no significant differences have been reported in systolic or diastolic blood pressure, serum sodium, serum potassium, fractional excretion of sodium, or transtubular potassium gradient between affected individuals and their unaffected relatives. The elevated serum aldosterone level was the only biochemical marker of rPHA1. However, reports from several families suggest that adult carriers of *NR3C2* mutations might also have normal levels of aldosterone [23].

PHA Type 2

PHA2 is characterized by hyperkalemia and hypertension. It is also known as Gordon syndrome [24]. Gordon syndrome is a heterogeneous syndrome with highly variable plasma aldosterone concentrations combined with suppressed plasma renin activity, various degrees of hyperchloremia and metabolic acidosis. Thus, Gordon syndrome does not include all clinical features of PHA, although the inability of the kidney to secrete potassium in this condition reflects a certain degree of aldosterone resistance. Renal and adrenal functions are normal. PHA2 shows an autosomal dominant mode of inheritance. As reflected in the variable clinical phenotype, the disease is linked to at least four genetic loci, including chromosomes 1, 12, 16 and 17. Deletions and mutations of two members of the WNK serine-threonine kinase family (WNK1 and WNK4) were identified in Gordon syndrome [25]. All subtypes of Gordon syndrome can be treated with low doses of thiazide diuretics which ameliorate all clinical findings.

PHA Type 3

PHA3 subsumes transient and secondary forms of salt-losing diseases caused by different pathologies related to kidney, intestine or sweat glands. Urinary tract infections and obstructive uropathies are the most frequent cause [26]. Contrary to PHA1 and PHA2, the glomerular filtration rate is decreased in these cases. The mechanism resulting in transient mineralocorticoid resistance is not clear. Salt losing episodes resulting from major intestine resection or sweat gland dysfunction are extremely rare.

Conclusion

PHA1 is a potentially life-threatening salt losing disease manifesting in neonates and infants. The systemic form is persisting in adulthood, whereas the salt loss in the renal form ameliorates during childhood. PHA1 is a state of mineralocorticoid resistance caused by inactivating mutations in the ENaC subunit genes in the case of sPHA1 or by inactivating mutations in the MR coding gene in the case of rPHA1. The latest reports suggest that an overlap of phenotypes due to partially inactivating ENaC inactivations seems to be possible. However, due to the rarity of the disease, the clinical descriptions and investigations available do not allow to conclude whether there is a genotype-phenotype correlation beyond the categories of sPHA1 and rPHA1. Therefore, future studies focusing on the clinical workup of the disease are warranted.

References

1 Arriza JL, Weinberger C, Cerelli G, Glaser TM, Handelin BL, Housman DE, Evans RM: Cloning of human mineralocorticoid receptor complementary DNA: structural and functional kinship with the glucocorticoid receptor. Science 1987;237:268–275.

2 Rogerson FM, Fuller PJ: Interdomain interactions in the mineralocorticoid receptor. Mol Cell Endocrinol 2003;200:45–55.

3 Fagart J, Huyet J, Pinon GM, Rochel M, Mayer C, Rafestin-Oblin ME: Crystal structure of a mutant mineralocorticoid receptor responsible for hypertension. Nat Struct Mol Biol 2005;12:554–555.

4 Garty H, Palmer LG: Epithelial sodium channels: function, structure, and regulation. Physiol Rev 1997;77:359–396.

5 Jasti J, Furukawa H, Gonzales EB, Gouaux E: Structure of acid-sensing ion channel 1 at 1.9 a resolution and low pH. Nature 2007;449:316–323.

6 Staub O, Gautschi I, Ishikawa T, Breitschopf K, Ciechanover A, Schild L, Rotin D: Regulation of stability and function of the epithelial Na^+ channel (ENaC) by ubiquitination. EMBO J 1997;16:6325–6336.

7 Fuller PJ, Young MJ: Mechanisms of mineralocorticoid action. Hypertension 2005;46:1227–1235.

8 Pearce D, Bhargava A, Cole TJ: Aldosterone: its receptor, target genes, and actions. Vitam Horm 2003;66:29–76.

9 Pearce D: SGK1 regulation of epithelial sodium transport. Cell Physiol Biochem 2003;13:13–20.

10 Spindler B, Verrey F: Aldosterone action: induction of p21(ras) and fra-2 and transcription-independent decrease in myc, jun, and fos. Am J Physiol 1999; 276:C1154–C1161.

11 Park J, Leong ML, Buse P, Maiyar AC, Firestone GL, Hemmings BA: Serum and glucocorticoid-inducible kinase (SGK) is a target of the PI 3-kinase-stimulated signaling pathway. EMBO J 1999;18:3024–3033.

12 Bhalla V, Daidie D, Li H, Pao AC, LaGrange LP, Wang J, Vandewalle A, Stockand JD, Staub O, Pearce D: Serum- and glucocorticoid-regulated kinase 1 regulates ubiquitin ligase neural precursor cell-expressed, developmentally down-regulated protein 4-2 by inducing interaction with 14-3-3. Mol Endocrinol 2005;19:3073–3084.

13 Cheek D, Perry J: A salt wasting syndrome in infancy. Arch Dis Child 1958;33:252–256.

14 Zennaro MC, Lombes M: Mineralocorticoid resistance. Trends Endocrinol Metab 2004;15:264–270.

15 Kerem E, Bistritzer T, Hanukoglu A, Hofmann T, Zhou Z, Bennett W, MacLaughlin E, Barker P, Nash M, Quittell L, Boucher R, Knowles MR: Pulmonary epithelial sodium-channel dysfunction and excess airway liquid in pseudohypoaldosteronism. N Engl J Med 1999;341:156–162.

16 Chang SS, Grunder S, Hanukoglu A, Rosler A, Mathew PM, Hanukoglu I, Schild L, Lu Y, Shimkets RA, Nelson-Williams C, Rossier BC, Lifton RP: Mutations in subunits of the epithelial sodium channel cause salt wasting with hyperkalaemic acidosis, pseudohypoaldosteronism type 1. Nat Genet 1996;12:248–253.

17 Dirlewanger M, Huser D, Zennaro MC, Girardin E, Schild L, Schwitzgebel VM: A homozygous missense mutation in SCNN1A is responsible for a transient neonatal form of pseudohypoaldosteronism type 1. Am J Physiol Endocrinol Metab 2011; 301:E467–E473.

18 Geller DS: Mineralocorticoid resistance. Clin Endocrinol (Oxf) 2005;62:513–520.

19 Geller DS, Rodriguez-Soriano J, Vallo Boado A, Schifter S, Bayer M, Chang SS, Lifton RP: Mutations in the mineralocorticoid receptor gene cause autosomal dominant pseudohypoaldosteronism type I. Nat Genet 1998;19:279–281.

20 Hanukoglu A, Joy O, Steinitz M, Rosler A, Hanukoglu I: Pseudohypoaldosteronism due to renal and multisystem resistance to mineralocorticoids respond differently to carbenoxolone. J Steroid Biochem Mol Biol 1997;60:105–112.

21 Riepe FG, Finkeldei J, de Sanctis L, Einaudi S, Testa A, Karges B, Peter M, Viemann M, Grotzinger J, Sippell WG, Fejes-Toth G, Krone N: Elucidating the underlying molecular pathogenesis of NR3C2 mutants causing autosomal dominant pseudohypoaldosteronism type 1. J Clin Endocrinol Metab 2006;91:4552–4561.
22 Geller DS, Zhang J, Zennaro MC, Vallo-Boado A, Rodriguez-Soriano J, Furu L, Haws R, Metzger D, Botelho B, Karaviti L, Haqq AM, Corey H, Janssens S, Corvol P, Lifton RP: Autosomal dominant pseudohypoaldosteronism type 1: mechanisms, evidence for neonatal lethality, and phenotypic expression in adults. J Am Soc Nephrol 2006;17: 1429–1436.
23 Riepe FG, Krone N, Morlot M, Peter M, Sippell WG, Partsch CJ: Autosomal-dominant pseudohypoaldosteronism type 1 in a Turkish family is associated with a novel nonsense mutation in the human mineralocorticoid receptor gene. J Clin Endocrinol Metab 2004;89:2150–2152.
24 Gordon RD: Syndrome of hypertension and hyperkalemia with normal glomerular filtration rate. Hypertension 1986;8:93–102.
25 Wilson FH, Disse-Nicodeme S, Choate KA, Ishikawa K, Nelson-Williams C, Desitter I, Gunel M, Milford DV, Lipkin GW, Achard JM, Feely MP, Dussol B, Berland Y, Unwin RJ, Mayan H, Simon DB, Farfel Z, Jeunemaitre X, Lifton RP: Human hypertension caused by mutations in WNK kinases. Science 2001;293:1107–1112.
26 Bulchmann G, Schuster T, Heger A, Kuhnle U, Joppich I, Schmidt H: Transient pseudohypoaldosteronism secondary to posterior urethral valves – a case report and review of the literature. Eur J Pediatr Surg 2001;11:277–279.

Felix G. Riepe, MD
Department of Pediatrics, Division of Pediatric Endocrinology
University Hospital Schleswig-Holstein
Schwanenweg 20, DE–24105 Kiel (Germany)
E-Mail friepe@pediatrics.uni-kiel.de

Maghnie M, Loche S, Cappa M, Ghizzoni L, Lorini R (eds): Hormone Resistance and Hypersensitivity. From Genetics to Clinical Management. Endocr Dev. Basel, Karger, 2013, vol 24, pp 96–105 (DOI: 10.1159/000342573)

New Aspects of the Physiology of the GH-IGF-1 Axis

Alessandra Vottero[a] · Chiara Guzzetti[b] · Sandro Loche[b]

[a]Clinica Pediatrica, Università di Parma, Parma, e [b]Servizio di Endocrinologia Pediatrica, Ospedale Regionale per le Microcitemie, ASL Cagliari, Cagliari, Italia

Abstract

Growth hormone (GH) secretion from the pituitary is regulated by a complex network of CNS and peripheral inputs. Circulating GH binds to its receptor and initiates a cascade of signaling events which involve the JAK2-STAT pathway, the PI3K/Akt pathway and the RAS/MAPK pathway, leading to the transcription of several genes, including insulin-like growth factor 1 (IGF-1), IGFBP3, ALS, and others. Recent findings indicate that nutrition plays an important role in GH secretion and action. Furthermore, data are emerging which suggest that the RAS-MAPK pathway as well as epigenetic regulation of transcription may be important in determining both circulating and locally produced IGF-1.

Evans and Long [1] identified the growth hormone (GH) about 75 years ago, but only in the last 20 years have the mechanisms underlying its actions been elucidated. The focus of this review is to discuss some of the latest findings on the physiology of GH secretion and action.

GH Receptor Structure

The GH receptor (GHR) was the first type I cytokine receptor cloned. It is a single-chain membrane-spanning protein consisting of an extracellular domain (ECD), a transmembrane domain, and an intracellular domain (ICD). The ECD is formed by two fibronectin type III β-sandwich domains connected to a rigid single-pass helical transmembrane domain via a flexible linker. The ICD comprises Box 1 and Box 2 motifs, which bind the tyrosine kinase JAK2, and several tyrosine residues that are substrates for phosphorylation by JAK2 [2].

GHR Mechanism of Action

GH, a 192-amino acid peptide secreted by the anterior pituitary, has pleiotropic effects on many tissues, including promoting somatic postnatal growth. GH is also an important metabolic hormone, partitioning nutrients into muscle and away from fat deposition, and together with insulin-like growth factor 1 (IGF-1) regulates bone turnover and chondrocyte proliferation [3]. Furthermore, it has many actions on hepatic metabolism, cardiac and immune function.

In the unbound state, GHR exists primarily as a homodimer. After binding to the hormone, the GHR undergoes some conformational changes and dimerizes promoting the transmission of the information through the cell membrane to the intracellular part of the GHR and leading to JAK2 activation and phosphorylation [4]. However, several data support the existence of a constitutive receptor dimer on the surface of the cell in the absence of GH [2]. A schematic representation of the GHR and the intracellular signaling machinery is shown in figure 1.

GH-IGF-1 Axis: New Aspects

The GH-IGF-1 system includes hypothalamic regulatory centers, the anterior pituitary gland, peripheral target organs, binding proteins, receptor and signaling molecules [5]. Responsiveness to GH in target cells is primarily dependent upon the expression of GHR [6].

Since class I cytokine receptors do not have intrinsic tyrosine kinase activity, they rely on associated tyrosine kinases for signal transduction. JAK2 associates with the GHR ICD proline-rich Box1 motif via its amino terminal (JH5–7) FERM domain and phosphorylates tyrosine residues on the associated GHR ICD. This phosphorylation provides docking sites for Src homology 2 (SH2) domain proteins STATS (signal transducers and activators of transcription), in particular STAT5a and -5b. STATs are phosphorylated by JAK2, homo- or heterodimerize, translocate to the nucleus, bind to STAT-responsive elements and activate transcription [2].

The unliganded GHR, in this particular conformation, autoinhibits the JH1 kinase domain and consequently inhibits JAK2. On the other hand, the constitutive dimer receptor causes a reorientation of JAK2 that disrupts the ability of pseudokinase JH2 to inhibit the JH1 kinase domain and therefore JAK2 is activated [2].

GHR is downregulated by several mechanisms including phosphatases, suppressors of cytokine signaling (SOCS) proteins and receptor downregulation, and ubiquitinization of the activated receptor [1]. Autophosphorylation of a site in the JAK2 FERM domain also inhibits receptor-mediated cytokine signaling [2].

Postnatal growth in humans is largely controlled by liver-derived IGF-1, whose gene transcription is STAT5b dependent. In particular, since early studies in the late 1990s [4], it became clear that STAT5b is the crucial signaling

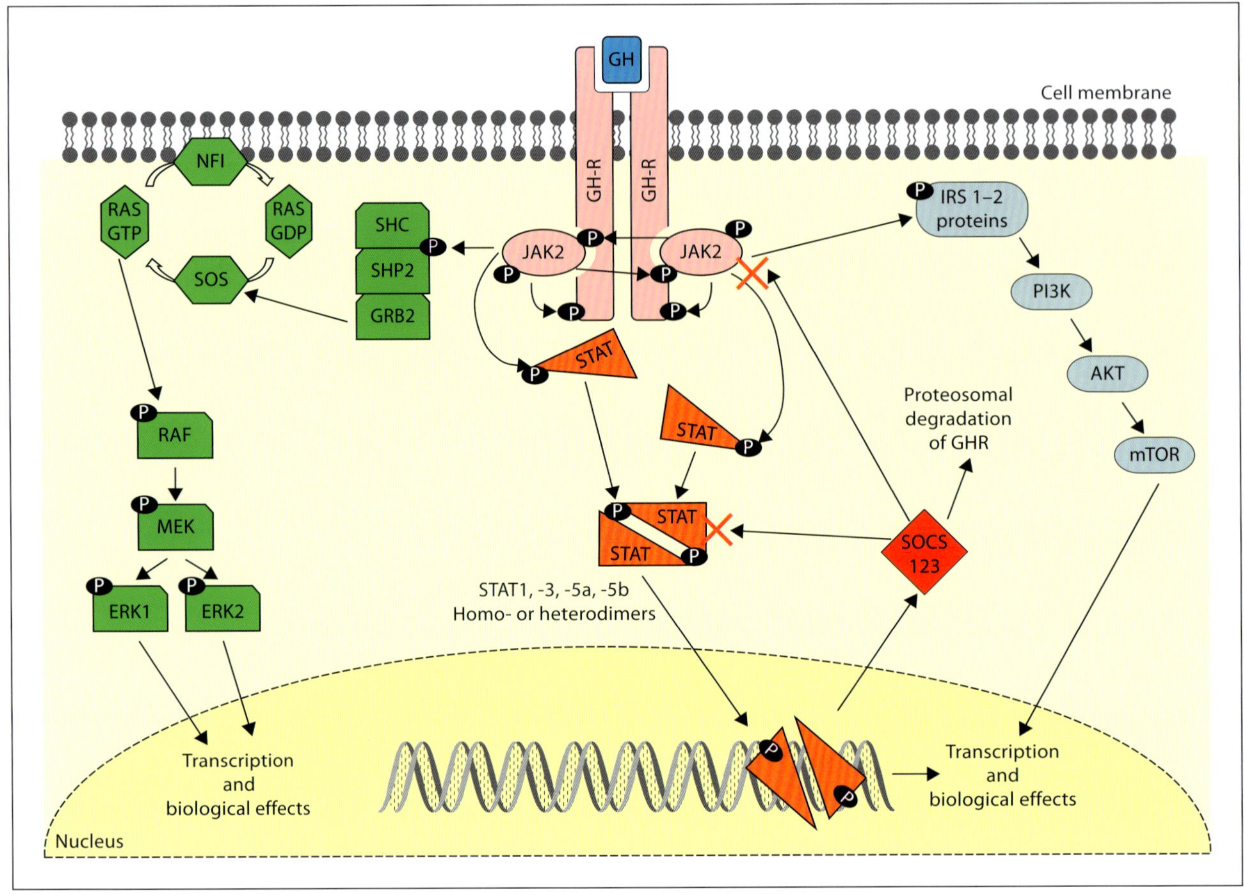

Fig. 1. Schematic representation of the GHR and intracellular signaling mechanism.

intermediate for GH-regulated growth. In particular, it is responsible for many of the long-term physiological actions of GH [7]. Its importance was confirmed by the discovery that mutations in the STA5b gene cause severe growth failure and short stature [8].

In mammals, the IGF-1 gene is composed of six exons and five introns that span more than 80 kb of chromosomal DNA. It contains two promoters, 1 and 2, of which the smaller promoter 2 is expressed mainly in the liver. Beyond the transcriptional control by these tandem promoters, IGF-1 mRNA undergoes alternative splicing involving exon 5 and 6, and polyadenylation at the 3′ end of exon 6, both of them generating over 100 distinct IGF-1 mRNAs. However, only the same 70-amino acid mature IGF-1 peptide is encoded. This is not completely understood, although different turnover and sensitivity of the IGF-1 mRNAs could be responsible for this phenomenon.

For a long time, it was believed that GHR was able to utilize only the JAK/STAT signaling pathway. However, new lines of evidence indicate that GHR signals through other JAK2-independent pathways. Barclay et al. [9] characterized mice in whom the JAK2-STAT5 signaling was abrogated while maintaining other signal pathways, and provided elegant evidence of GH-dependent activation of the Src family tyrosine kinase (SFK)/extracellular-regulated kinase (ERK) signaling pathway. The SFK is a signaling pathway independent of JAK2 which activates the ERKs 1 and 2 (p44/42 MAPK) [2, 9]. The Src kinase Lyn binds directly to the membrane proximal part of the GHR even in the absence of JAK2, independent of hormone binding. In particular, there is a rearrangement of a loop in the lower cytokine receptor module of the GHR that occurs when GH agonists, but not antagonists, are bound, and this rearrangement is necessary for activation of Src and ERK by the GHR in myeloid cells [9]. Mutations in several genes encoding proteins of the RAS-MAPK/ERK pathway cause a series of diseases also termed RASopathies, which include Noonan syndrome. About half of patients with Noonan syndrome carry a mutation in the PTPN11 gene encoding the tyrosine phosphatase SHP2 [10]. Patients with Noonan syndrome have growth retardation associated with low IGF-1 levels, which are even lower in the patients carrying the mutation [11, 12]. Recently, it has been shown that activating mutations of the tyrosine phosphate SHP2 in mice inhibit GH-induced IGF-1 release through RAS/ERK1/2 hyperactivation, contributing to growth retardation [13]. These findings shed new light not only on the mechanisms underlying growth retardation in different syndromes associated with short stature, but also on possible future treatment strategies to improve the outcome of patients with poor responses to conventional GH therapy [14].

In order to avoid excessive and off-target effects secondary to GHR activation, target tissue responsiveness to GH is downregulated. In particular, the SOCS2 is a key regulator of GHR sensitivity [15]. Studies in mice demonstrated that SOCS2 is an important negative regulator of GHR signaling since SOCS2-deficient mice show a 40% increase in body size due to enhanced postnatal growth [16]. Furthermore, SOCS2 has been recently shown to be a critical regulator of GH action in the mouse growth plate chondrogenesis [17]. The negative feedback loop operated by SOCS2 involves GH-activated Stat5b which binds to the promoter of SOCS2 promoting its expression and, in turn, SOCS2 binds to at least two phosphorylated tyrosines on the GHR to negatively regulate JAK2 and Stat5b activation. However, the exact underlying biochemical mechanism is still not completely elucidated and might include the lack of binding to positive regulators [18] and/or the interaction with proteins for proteosomal degradation [18]. Vesterlund et al. [18] showed that SOCS2 is part of a multimeric complex with intrinsic ubiquitin ligase activity including Cullin5, Rbx2, and elongins C and B. The SOCS2 ubiquitin ligase complex has the ability to ubiquitinate the GHR in vitro and downregulate GHR in a proteasomally dependent manner, mediated by both a functional

SOCS box and its interaction with Tyr487 in the ICD of the GHR. The SOCS box is very important for the proper function of SOCS2, and it is located at the C-terminus end of the protein, similarly to other ubiquitin ligases. Deletion of the SOCS-box abrogates the inhibitory actions of SOCS2 on GH-induced Stat5b activation [18].

Genome-wide association studies identified SOCS2 as one of the 20 loci that influence human adult height [19]. Many polymorphisms in the SOCS2 gene were also identified in humans, one linked to height [19]. Furthermore, SOCS proteins may also be involved in the growth retardation that accompanies many chronic diseases such as inflammatory bowel disease or rheumatoid arthritis [20].

Factors Influencing the GH-IGF-1 Axis: Nutrition and Epigenetics

Nutrition

GH secretion is regulated by the coordinate action of GH-releasing hormone and somatostatin which, respectively, stimulate and inhibit its release from the pituitary. The release of these two hypothalamic neurohormones is, in turn, regulated by a complex network of neurotransmitters and neuropeptides. GH secretion is also regulated by a feedback mechanism by itself and by IGF-1 which exert their negative effect on both the hypothalamus and the pituitary. Other hormones including sex steroids, glucocorticoids, gastrointestinal hormones as well as metabolic fuels participate in GH regulation. The net result of this complex regulation is an episodic secretion of GH, which increases during sleep. Evaluation of GH secretion, thus, cannot be performed by measuring GH in a random serum sample. Stimulation tests have been used for decades for evaluating GH secretory status, although they are poorly reproducible, inaccurate, and yield a considerable number of false-positive responses also in normal children [21]. Furthermore, the great majority of children with a biochemical diagnosis of isolated idiopathic GH deficiency show normalization of GH secretion when retested after months or years [22, 23]. There are a number of reasons which may explain this variability [21]. Nutrition and metabolism play a key role in the regulation of the GH-IGF-1 pathway, and adults and children with nutritional problems show profound modifications of the GH-IGF-1 axis. Subjects with anorexia have increased GH secretion and reduced IGF-1 serum levels, indicating GH resistance [24]. On the other hand, obese children have normal-high serum IGF-1 levels, associated with reduced spontaneous and stimulated GH secretion [25], indicating an increase in GH responsiveness [26, 27]. In obesity, stimulated GH peak is negatively correlated with BMI [25]. Furthermore, both fasting [28] and overfeeding also have acute effects on GH secretion [29]. More recently, it has been demonstrated that BMI has

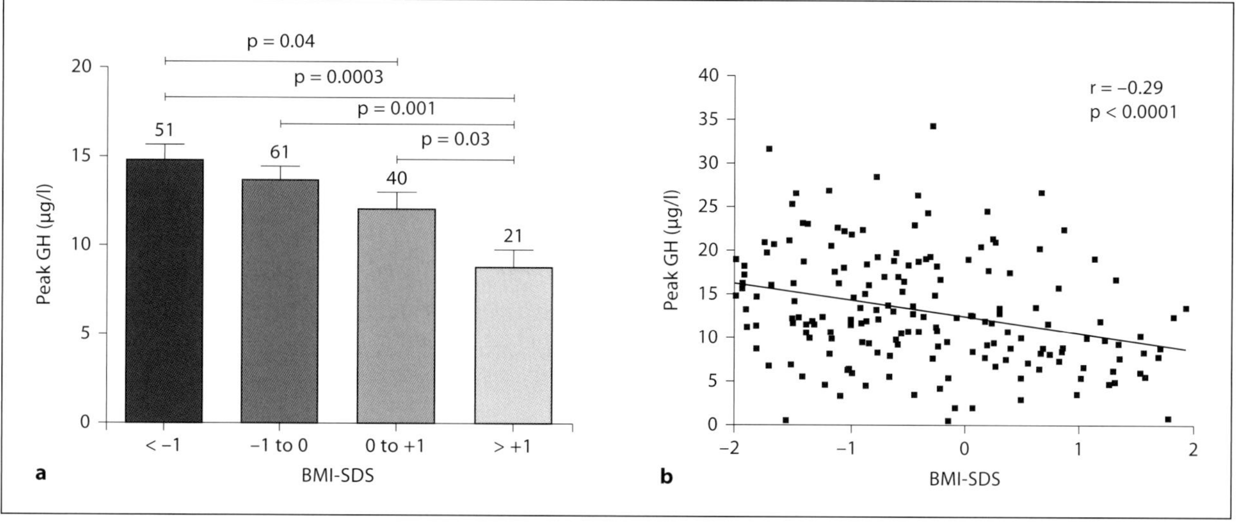

Fig. 2. a Peak GH (mean ± SE) after clonidine testing in 173 short children subdivided according to BMI-SDS. The number of subjects in each group is shown in the columns. **b** Correlation between the peak GH after clonidine testing and BMI-SDS.

a considerable impact on GH secretion in children over a wide range of BMI and after various stimulation tests, indicating that BMI (and hence nutrition) may be one of the most important factors influencing the variability of the GH responses to stimulation tests [30–32] (fig. 2).

The importance of these findings in the clinical setting is obvious since a number of children and adults may be falsely diagnosed as GHD [33]. Even mild elevation of BMI determines a reduced GH response, strongly contributing to the variability of the magnitude of peak GH. Based on these observations, recently, different cut-off GH values according to the BMI were proposed for the combined arginine + GH-releasing hormone stimulation test [34, 35] to increase its specificity in adult subjects.

The pathogenesis of this phenomenon is still not clear, and appears to be multifactorial, including the contribution of insulin, circulating free fatty acids, and also leptin [25]. Fibroblast growth factor 21 (FGF21), a recently identified metabolic hormone, has been shown to function as a physiological mediator of the effects of severe food deprivation on the GH-IGF-1 axis [36]. Inhibition of IGF-1 gene expression and blunted somatic growth have been demonstrated in mice overexpressing FGF21 through a mechanism involving reduction of STAT5b phosphorylation [4]. FGF21 may also participate in a GH-activated negative feedback loop since its expression is induced indirectly by the acute metabolic actions of GH on adipocytes [4].

Epigenetics

Preliminary data from the Epigrow Study [37] have shown that more that 50% of short children with normal GH responses to stimulation have subnormal IGF-1 concentrations. This finding suggests that something in the GH signaling machine might not function properly. In fact, although Stat5b is the critical intracellular mediator of GH action, including IGF-1 gene transcription, the molecular mechanisms by which GH-activated Stat5b promotes IGF-1 gene activity is not entirely known [4]. Furthermore, unlike several other GH-responsive and Stat5b-regulated genes [4], the IGF-1 gene lacks specific promoter-associated Stat5b response elements. Only a Sta5-binding DNA segment, called HS7, was mapped in the proximity of the two promoters, specifically in intron 2 about 1.6 kb 3′ to exon 2.

Two recent reports [38, 39] have shown that gene transcription induced by GH is accompanied by acute chromatin changes. These epigenetic modifications include immediate stimulation of core histone acetylation and modifications in histone methylation. This results in IGF-1 gene transcription activation in the liver by distinct promoter-specific mechanisms. At IGF-1 promoter 1, GH causes RNA Pol II to be released from a previously recruited paused preinitiation complex, whereas at promoter 2, hormone treatment facilitates recruitment and then activation of RNA Pol II to initiate transcription. These modifications make the chromosomal DNA more accessible to transcription factors and other regulatory proteins typically involved in signal-mediated gene activation.

Therefore, GH exerts dramatic and variable epigenetic actions on genes that are acutely regulated by Stat5b, such as SOCS2, Cish, Igfals, and Spi 2.1, which share a very similar genomic architecture. More studies are needed to better define the dynamics of the epigenetic changes induced by GH under physiological and pathological conditions, but open a new window to the complexity of GH action.

Conclusions

In the last decades, a number of important findings have contributed to the understanding of the physiology of the GH-IGF-1 axis. It is now well known that Stat5b is the crucial intracellular mediator of GH action. The active Stat5b interacts with multiple binding sites in chromatin within the IGF-1 locus and, through mechanisms not fully characterized, promotes the transmission of signal to the two IGF-1 promoters. This results in the induction of IGF-1 gene transcription and the production of IGF-1 mRNAs and protein. This is the leading pathway involved in postnatal growth and, in fact, its medical significance was confirmed by identification of inactivating Stat5b mutations in children with profound GH-resistant growth failure. However, GH-mediated IGF-1 gene regulation is extremely complex both in physiologic and pathologic conditions, and still not completely known.

In humans, GH secretion is under the control of several metabolic factors, and it is influenced by age, sex, circulating hormone levels, and nutritional status. Recent studies in adults and children have shown that nutrition plays an important role in the regulation of GH secretion. These studies have shown consistently that BMI is significantly and negatively correlated with GH secretion. The mechanisms underlying the role of nutrition/BMI on GH secretion, and the causative factors and metabolic consequences of reduced GH with increasing adiposity are still not clear and deserve further studies.

Epigenetic regulation of GH-induced gene activation is emerging as another important step in controlling IGF-1 synthesis and secretion. It was predicted that exogenous and endogenous hormonal pulses induce a rapid chromatin modification at the IGF-1 promoters involving acetylation and deacetylation, methylation and demethylation of core histones, together with the recruitment and modification of transcriptional coregulators which represent fundamental and physiologically relevant dynamic genomic effects of GH. The connection between activation of Stat5b and the nuclear events culminating in acute chromatin reorganization and induction of IGF-1 gene transcription remains to be clarified.

References

1 Waters MJ, Hoang HN, Fairlie DP, Pelekanos RA, Brown RJ: New insights into growth hormone action. J Mol Endocrinol 2006;36:1–7.
2 Brooks AJ, Wooh JW, Tunny KA, Waters MJ: Growth hormone receptor; mechanism of action. Int J Biochem Cell Biol 2008;40:1984–1989.
3 Waters MJ, Brooks AJ: Growth hormone receptor: structure function relationships. Horm Res Paediatr 2011;(suppl 1):12–16.
4 Rotwein P: Mapping the growth hormone – Stat5b-IGF-I transcriptional circuit. Trends Endocrinol Metab 2012;23:186–193.
5 Veldhuis JD, Roemmich JN, Richmond EJ, Bowers CY: Somatotropic and gonadotropic axes linkages in infancy, childhood, and the puberty-adult transition. Endocr Rev 2006;27:101–140.
6 Flores-Morales A, Greenhalgh CJ, Norstedt G, Rico-Bautista E: Negative regulation of growth hormone receptor signaling. Mol Endocrinol 2006; 20:241–253.
7 Rotwein P, Chia DJ: Gene regulation by growth hormone. Pediatr Nephrol 2010;25:651–658.
8 Hwa V, Nadeau K, Wit JM, Rosenfeld RG: STAT5b deficiency: lessons from STAT5b gene mutations. Best Pract Res Clin Endocrinol Metab 2011;25: 61–75.
9 Barclay JL, Kerr LM, Arthur L, Rowland JE, Nelson CN, Ishikawa M, d'Aniello EM, White M, Noakes PG, Waters MJ: In vivo targeting of the growth hormone receptor (GHR) Box1 sequence demonstrates that the GHR does not signal exclusively through JAK2. Mol Endocrinol 2010;24: 204–217.
10 Tartaglia M, Kalidas K, Shaw A, Song X, Musat DL, van dB, I, Brunner HG, Bertola DR, Crosby A, Ion A, Kucherlapati RS, Jeffery S, Patton MA, Gelb BD: PTPN11 mutations in Noonan syndrome: molecular spectrum, genotype-phenotype correlation, and phenotypic heterogeneity. Am J Hum Genet 2002; 70:1555–1563.
11 Limal JM, Parfait B, Cabrol S, Bonnet D, Leheup B, Lyonnet S, Vidaud M, Le BY: Noonan syndrome: relationships between genotype, growth, and growth factors. J Clin Endocrinol Metab 2006; 91:300–306.
12 Binder G, Neuer K, Ranke MB, Wittekindt NE: PTPN11 mutations are associated with mild growth hormone resistance in individuals with Noonan syndrome. J Clin Endocrinol Metab 2005;90:5377–5381.

13 De Rocca Serra-Nédélec A, Edouard T, Treguer K, Tajan M, Araki T, Dance M, Mus M, Montagner A, Tauber M, Salles JP, Valet P, Neel BG, Raynal P, Yart A: Noonan syndrome-causing SHP2 mutants inhibit insulin-like growth factor 1 release via growth hormone-induced ERK hyperactivation, which contributes to short stature. Proc Natl Acad Sci U S A 2012;109:4257–4262.

14 Wu X, Simpson J, Hong JH, Kim KH, Thavarajah NK, Backx PH, Neel BG, Araki T: MEK-ERK pathway modulation ameliorates disease phenotypes in a mouse model of Noonan syndrome associated with the Raf1(L613V) mutation. J Clin Invest 2011; 121:1009–1025.

15 Greenhalgh CJ, Alexander WS: Suppressors of cytokine signalling and regulation of growth hormone action. Growth Horm IGF Res 2004;14:200–206.

16 Greenhalgh CJ, Rico-Bautista E, Lorentzon M, Thaus AL, Morgan PO, Willson TA, Zervoudakis P, Metcalf D, Street I, Nicola NA, Nash AD, Fabri LJ, Norstedt G, Ohlsson C, Flores-Morales A, Alexander WS, Hilton DJ: SOCS2 negatively regulates growth hormone action in vitro and in vivo. J Clin Invest 2005;115:397–406.

17 Pass C, Macrae VE, Huesa C, Ahmed SF, Farquharson C: SOCS2 is the critical regulator of GH action in murine growth plate chondrogenesis. J Bone Miner Res 2012;27:1055–1066.

18 Vesterlund M, Zadjali F, Persson T, Nielsen ML, Kessler BM, Norstedt G, Flores-Morales A: The SOCS2 ubiquitin ligase complex regulates growth hormone receptor levels. PLoS One 2011;6:e25358.

19 Weedon MN, Lango H, Lindgren CM, et al: Genome-wide association analysis identifies 20 loci that influence adult height. Nat Genet 2008;40: 575–583.

20 Ahmed SF, Farquharson C: The effect of GH and IGF1 on linear growth and skeletal development and their modulation by SOCS proteins. J Endocrinol 2010;206:249–259.

21 Cappa M, Loche S: Evaluation of growth disorders in the paediatric clinic. J Endocrinol Invest 2003; 26:54–63.

22 Loche S, Bizzarri C, Maghnie M, Faedda A, Tzialla C, Autelli M, Casini MR, Cappa M: Results of early reevaluation of growth hormone secretion in short children with apparent growth hormone deficiency. J Pediatr 2002;140:445–449.

23 Maghnie M, Strigazzi C, Tinelli C, Autelli M, Cisternino M, Loche S, Severi F: Growth hormone (GH) deficiency (GHD) of childhood onset: reassessment of GH status and evaluation of the predictive criteria for permanent GHD in young adults. J Clin Endocrinol Metab 1999;84:1324–1328.

24 Miller KK: Endocrine dysregulation in anorexia nervosa update. J Clin Endocrinol Metab 2011;96: 2939–2949.

25 Kreitschmann-Andermahr I, Suarez P, Jennings R, Evers N, Brabant G: GH/IGF-I regulation in obesity – mechanisms and practical consequences in children and adults. Horm Res Paediatr 2010;73: 153–160.

26 Bouhours-Nouet N, Gatelais F, Boux de CF, Rouleau S, Coutant R: The insulin-like growth factor-I response to growth hormone is increased in prepubertal children with obesity and tall stature. J Clin Endocrinol Metab 2007;92:629–635.

27 Gleeson HK, Lissett CA, Shalet SM: Insulin-like growth factor-I response to a single bolus of growth hormone is increased in obesity. J Clin Endocrinol Metab 2005;90:1061–1067.

28 Ho KY, Veldhuis JD, Johnson ML, Furlanetto R, Evans WS, Alberti KG, Thorner MO: Fasting enhances growth hormone secretion and amplifies the complex rhythms of growth hormone secretion in man. J Clin Invest 1988;81:968–975.

29 Cornford AS, Barkan AL, Horowitz JF: Rapid suppression of growth hormone concentration by overeating: potential mediation by hyperinsulinemia. J Clin Endocrinol Metab 2011;96:824–830.

30 Stanley TL, Levitsky LL, Grinspoon SK, Misra M: Effect of body mass index on peak growth hormone response to provocative testing in children with short stature. J Clin Endocrinol Metab 2009;94: 4875–4881.

31 Lee HS, Hwang JS: Influence of body mass index on growth hormone responses to classic provocative tests in children with short stature. Neuroendocrinology 2011;93:259–264.

32 Loche S, Guzzetti C, Pilia S, Ibba A, Civolani P, Porcu M, Minerba L, Casini MR: Effect of body mass index on the growth hormone response to clonidine stimulation testing in children with short stature. Clin Endocrinol (Oxf) 2011;74:726–731.

33 Bonert VS, Elashoff JD, Barnett P, Melmed S: Body mass index determines evoked growth hormone (GH) responsiveness in normal healthy male subjects: diagnostic caveat for adult GH deficiency. J Clin Endocrinol Metab 2004;89:3397–3401.

34 Corneli G, Di SC, Baldelli R, Rovere S, Gasco V, Croce CG, Grottoli S, Maccario M, Colao A, Lombardi G, Ghigo E, Camanni F, Aimaretti G: The cutoff limits of the GH response to GH-releasing hormone-arginine test related to body mass index. Eur J Endocrinol 2005;153:257–264.

35 Colao A, Di SC, Savastano S, Rota F, Savanelli MC, Aimaretti G, Lombardi G: A reappraisal of diagnosing GH deficiency in adults: role of gender, age, waist circumference, and body mass index. J Clin Endocrinol Metab 2009;94:4414–4422.
36 Fazeli PK, Misra M, Goldstein M, Miller KK, Klibanski A: Fibroblast growth factor-21 may mediate growth hormone resistance in anorexia nervosa. J Clin Endocrinol Metab 2010;95:369–374.
37 Clayton P, Maisonobe P, Dutailly P: High prevalence of insulin-like growth factor-I deficiency in idiopathic short stature children. Endocr Rev 2011; 32:P1–725.
38 Chia DJ, Young JJ, Mertens AR, Rotwein P: Distinct alterations in chromatin organization of the two IGF-I promoters precede growth hormone-induced activation of IGF-I gene transcription. Mol Endocrinol 2010;24:779–789.
39 Chia DJ, Rotwein P: Defining the epigenetic actions of growth hormone: acute chromatin changes accompany GH-activated gene transcription. Mol Endocrinol 2010;24:2038–2049.

Dr. Sandro Loche
Servizio di Endocrinologia Pediatrica, Ospedale Regionale per le Microcitemie
Via Jenner snc
IT–09121 Cagliari (Italy)
E-Mail sandroloche@asl8cagliari.it

Maghnie M, Loche S, Cappa M, Ghizzoni L, Lorini R (eds): Hormone Resistance and Hypersensitivity. From Genetics to Clinical Management. Endocr Dev. Basel, Karger, 2013, vol 24, pp 106–117 (DOI: 10.1159/000342575)

Molecular and Clinical Aspects of GHRH Receptor Mutations

Valentina Corazzini · Roberto Salvatori

Division of Endocrinology and Metabolism, School of Medicine, Johns Hopkins University, Baltimore, Md., USA

Abstract

The growth hormone (GH)-releasing hormone (GHRH) receptor (GHRHR) belongs to the G protein-coupled receptor family. It binds GHRH resulting in somatotroph cell proliferation and stimulation of GH secretion. Mutations in the gene encoding for GHRHR (*GHRHR*, OMIM No. 139191) are being reported with increasing frequency in familial isolated GH deficiency. To date, the reported *GHRHR* mutations include eight missense, seven splice, three microdeletions, and two non-sense mutations. One promoter mutation has also been reported. Most of these mutations show a recessive mode of inheritance. The phenotype includes reduced but not absent serum GH, with abnormal response to a variety of stimuli, and low serum insulin-like growth factor-1 levels, resulting in proportionate growth failure which becomes evident in the first year of life. These patients respond well to GH replacement therapy. Phenotypical observations coming from some unusually large kindreds with untreated GH deficiency due to homozygous *GHRHR* mutations have allowed the study of the consequences of lifetime lack of GH. This chapter reviews the structure and the role of the GHRHR together with the clinical aspects associated with its mutations.

Growth hormone (GH) is the most important regulator of linear growth. GH secretion by the somatotroph cells of the anterior pituitary gland is under control of multiple hormonal agents including GH-releasing hormone (GHRH), ghrelin, and somatostatin. The former two exert stimulatory effects, while the latter one induces inhibition of somatotroph cell function. Deficiency in GH circulating levels causes postnatal somatic growth failure and metabolic alterations. Short stature caused by isolated GH deficiency (IGHD) has been estimated to occur in 1/4,000 to 1/10,000 live births. The majority of the cases can be associated with sporadic events like cerebral insults or abnormalities of the hypothalamic-pituitary region, and about 12% of cases show clear structural defects by magnetic resonance imaging (MRI). However, more than a quarter of the IGHD cases have a familial occurrence, supporting the hypothesis of a genetic cause [1]. Familial IGHD is traditionally classified into four classes based on the mode of inheritance, the clinical features, and the response to therapy. Type IA and IB are both autosomal recessive forms that differ in serum GH levels (undetectable in the first type, low but detectable in the second one) and treatment response (type IA patients often develop anti-GH antibodies after GH replacement). Type II is a form of IGHD with an autosomal dominant inheritance in which patients usually have low serum GH levels and no development of anti-GH antibodies. Occasionally, with time, these patients present additional pituitary hormone deficits. Finally, type III is a very rare X-linked form mainly associated with X-linked hypogammaglobulinemia [2]. GH gene *(GH-1)* mutations represent the principal genetic cause of type I and type II IGHD, but cause less than 2% of type IB cases, suggesting the involvement of different genes [1]. Owing to its important role in GH secretion, the GHRH gene was suspected to be involved in IGHD pathogenesis, but no mutations have been detected yet, whereas mutations in GHRH receptor (GHRHR) gene (*GHRHR)* have been reported with increasing frequency during the last decade.

GHRH and GHRHR: Physiology, Structure and Regulation

GHRH is a 44-amino acid peptide hormone produced mainly in the hypothalamus which is structurally related to the family of 'brain-gut' peptides including glucagon, glucagon-like peptide (GLP-1), vasoactive intestinal peptide (VIP), secretin, vasoactive intestinal polypeptide and pituitary adenylyl cyclase-activating peptide (PACAP) [3]. It was identified in 1982 in 2 patients affected by pancreatic tumors causing acromegaly, and then characterized from the hypothalamus. GHRH is first detectable in blood between 18 and 26 weeks of gestation, then levels become maximum in term human newborns and gradually decline after puberty [4]. GHRH is released from neurosecretory nerve terminals of arcuate neurons, and through the hypothalamo-hypophyseal portal system reaches the anterior pituitary gland where it binds to the GHRHR of the somatotroph cells causing both GH secretion and cell proliferation. The GHRHR is mostly expressed in the anterior pituitary gland, and it belongs to the family B, group III of the G protein-coupled receptor superfamily, including, among others, receptors for secretin, GLP-1, VIP and PACAP. The GHRHR consists of 423 amino acids with an N-terminal and a C-terminal portion linked by a 7-α-helice transmembrane (TM) domain. Part of the extracellular domain is cleaved after translation. The extracellular N-terminal domain contains an N-linked glycosylation site, and it does not exhibit high affinity for GHRH, but it is essential for ligand binding, the specificity of which is provided by the loops connecting the α-helices. The extracellular domain also influences the internalization of the protein. The C-terminal domain contains several potential phosphorylation sites and a cysteine that could undergo palmitoylation [4]. The binding of GHRH causes conformational changes in the receptor resulting in the activation of the $G_s\alpha$ subunit of the associated G protein complex, which in turn stimulates the membrane-bound adenylyl cyclase, causing the increase in intracellular cyclic

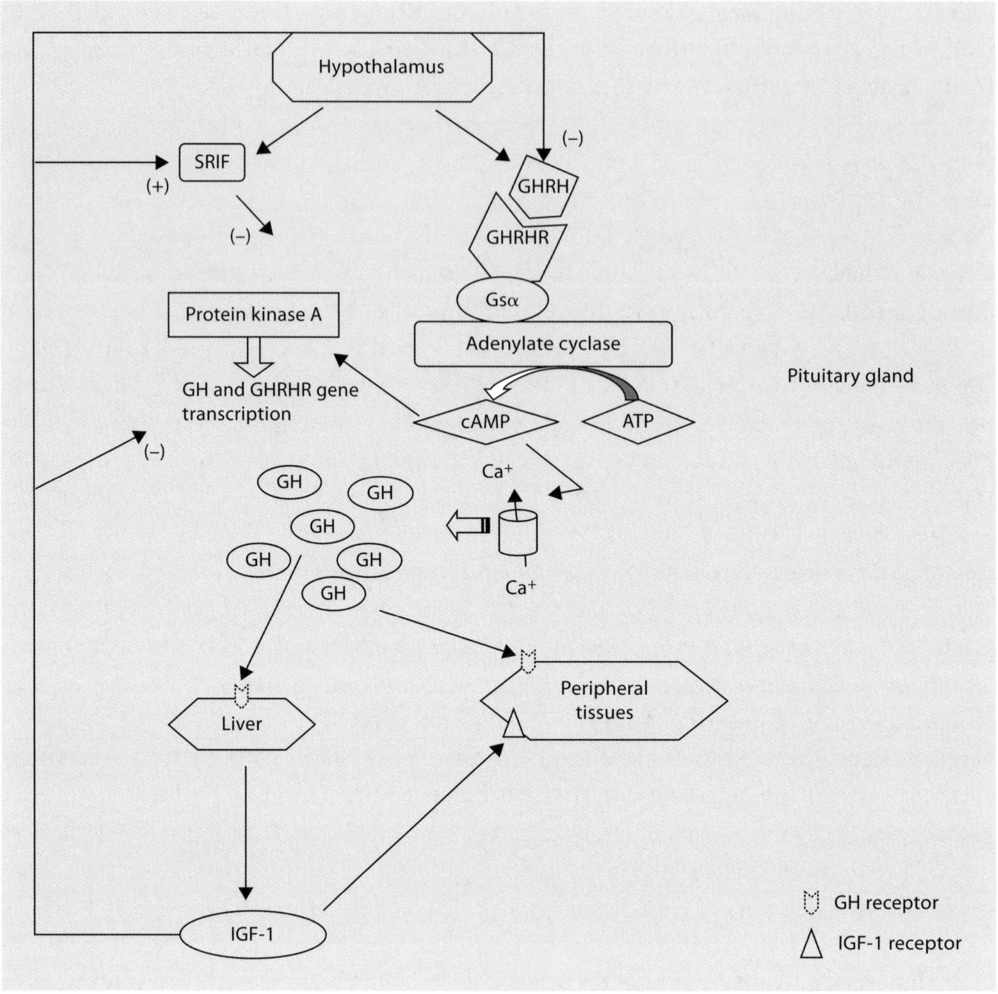

Fig. 1. Schematic representation of regulation of GH secretion by GHRH and of GH action.

adenosine monophosphate (cAMP) (fig. 1). cAMP activates the protein kinase A; this translocates to the nucleus and phosphorylates the transcription factor cAMP response element-binding protein (CREB). This, together with coactivators p300 and CREB-binding protein (CBP), is involved in the transcription of GH through a binding to CREs cAMP response elements in the target gene promoter region. This pattern increases transcription of the GHRHR gene, providing a positive feedback. Activation by GHRH causes also the opening of Na^+ channels by phosphatidylinositol 4,5-bisphosphate, and consequent cell depolarization. The resulting change in the intracellular voltage opens a voltage-dependent calcium channel, which causes vesicle fusion and release of GH [4]. Other transduction mechanisms have been involved, but they seem to play a minor role. As for all the G protein-coupled receptors, the GHRHR is also downregulated after activation: its overstimulation leads to the phosphorylation of different sites, resulting in the interaction of the receptor with the GRK/β-arrestin complex and in its silencing [2].

The GHRHR Gene

In humans, the GHRHR gene *(GHRHR)* is located on chromosome 7p143. It has a complex structure spanning about 15 kb and containing 13 exons. The expression of POU domain transcription pituitary-specific factor Pit-1 (POUF-1 according to the most recent nomenclature) is fundamental for transcription of the GHRHR gene in vivo. The 5′ flanking region of the gene contains several binding sites for other promoter regulatory factors such as CREB, the nuclear factor NF-1 and the upstream regulatory factor USF, the latter two known to bind also the GH gene promoter. The receptor's expression seems to be regulated mainly by GHRH itself via the CREB-binding site in the promoter region [4]. Glucocorticoids seem to have also an essential role in somatotroph differentiation during development and in GHRHR gene transcription, as demonstrated in adrenalectomized rats [5]. Thyroid-deficient state is associated with a decreased GHRHR gene expression [2], whereas estrogens have an inhibitory effect on GHRHR promoter that could explain the lower transcription levels in female compared to male rats at puberty. On the other hand, androgens directly increase GHRHR gene expression in the arcuate nucleus of the hypothalamus [5].

GHRH Gene Mutations

The first naturally occurring mouse model of inherited autosomal recessive GH-deficient dwarfism was serendipitously identified in 1970s at the Jackson Laboratories and named *little (lit/lit)* [6]. It was not until the 1990s that two different groups discovered that the dwarf phenotype of *lit* rodents is caused by a homozygous missense mutation in the GHRHR gene, a single base substitution (A>G) in codon 60 which encodes for an amino acid in the extracellular domain (D60G) affecting the ability of the receptor to bind GHRH [4]. This discovery triggered the search for *GHRHR* mutations in humans. The first mutation was described by Wajnrajch and colleagues in 1996, a G>T non-sense mutation in the extracellular domain (E72X) occurring in 2 IGHD cousins from a consanguineous Indian family. The same mutation was then reported in two villages in the province of Sindh in Pakistan [7] and in two siblings from Sri Lanka, and it soon became evident that it is highly prevalent in IGHD families from the Indian subcontinent [8], likely due to a 'founder effect'. However, very recently the same mutation has been reported in a Turkish kindred, which apparently has no Indian ancestry [9]. In 1999, we identified the largest kindred with autosomal recessive IGHD from Itabaianinha, in the northeastern Brazilian state of Sergipe. These 105 IGHD

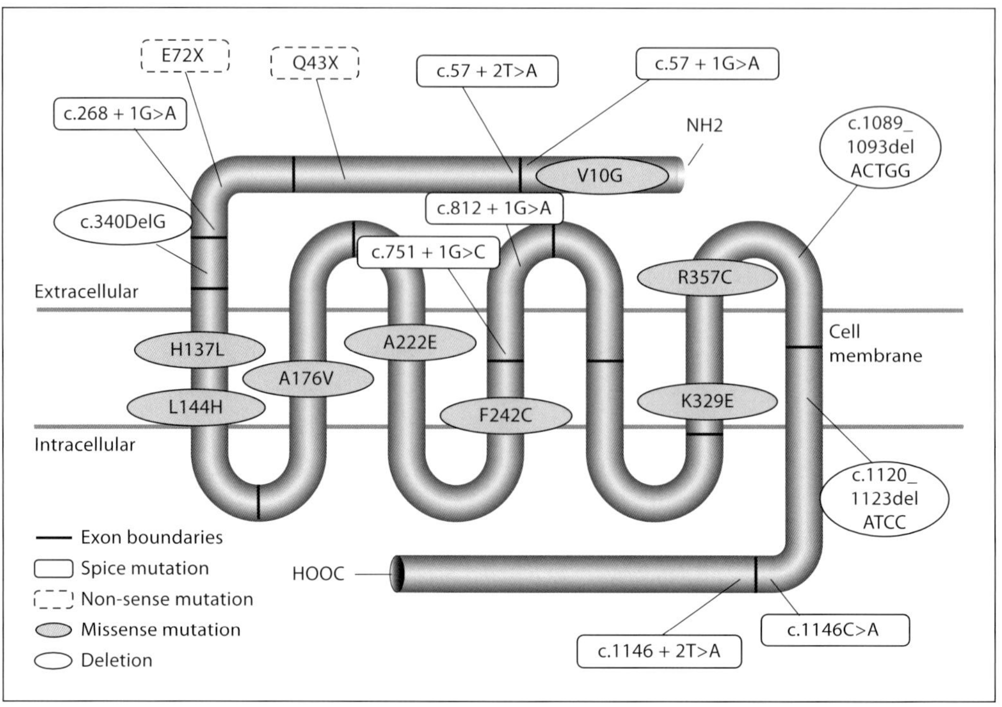

Fig. 2. Location of the GHRHR gene mutations. The promoter mutation is not represented here.

individuals through seven generations from the rural county of Itabaianinha have a homozygous mutation in the consensus GT of the 5′ splice site of intron 1, required for correct splicing of intron 1 from RNA transcripts (c.57 + 1G>A). This mutation likely leads to retention of intron 1 and insertion of a premature stop codon 213 bases from the exon-intron junction, similarly to what was later described for a different mutation in the same splice site [10]. A founder effect has been hypothesized in this population, in which the high incidence of consanguineous unions seems to be the principal cause for mutation spread [6]. Several *GHRHR* mutations have since then been described (fig. 2): six additional splice mutations (c.57 + 2T>A, c.268 + 1G>A, c.751 + 1G>C, c.812 + 1G>A, c.1146C>A, c.1146 + 2T>A), one non-sense mutation located in exon 2 (Q43X), eight missense mutations (V10G in exon 1, H137L and L144H in exon 5, A176V in exon 6, A222E and F242C in exon 7, K329E and R357C in exon 11), three deletions, one in exon 4 (c.340DelG) and two deletions in exon 11 (c.1089–1093delACTGG) and exon 12 (c.1120–1123delATCC) [1, 11–13]. Additionally, a mutation in the *GHRHR* promoter that impairs Pit1 binding and reduces gene expression has also been described (–124 A>C), bringing the total count to 21 mutations [2, 11]. Most *GHRHR* mutations seem to be specific to a single geographical area, with the exception of the L144H which has been reported in Spain, Brazil and USA, and for which linkage analysis suggests that it has arisen independently at least twice [11].

Regarding the mode of inheritance, most of the *GHRHR* mutations are inherited as autosomal recessive trait [2] with two exceptions. One, not fully proven, is represented by the c.1120–1123delATCC described in a heterozygous (HTZ) form in a severely GH-deficient Japanese boy. However, the patient was much shorter than his parents, seemingly contradicting this hypothesis [2]. Another exception, substantiated by in vitro studies, is represented by the V10G mutation described in 2009 by Godi et al. [13]. This amino acid change abolishes the cleavage of signal peptide from the mutant receptor which in turn is not translocated onto the cell surface. Because this mutation is present also in normal-stature relatives of the patients as well in normal controls, it could be a dominant mutation associated with incomplete penetrance.

While consanguinity is rather frequent in these kindreds, several cases have been reported of affected individuals who are compound heterozygotes for two distinct *GHRHR* mutations, suggesting that faulty *GHRHR* alleles may be rather prevalent in the general population.

All the microdeletions, the splice and the non-sense mutations are expected to produce an altered receptor causing the translation of a truncated or out of frame protein (if mRNA is translated at all, due to non-sense-mediated mRNA decay). The promoter mutation causes a reduced ability to bind Pit1 with a subsequent much lower transcriptional activity. Conversely, all the missense mutations, other than the V10G, cause substitution in amino acids that belong to one of the TM domains and lead to receptor malfunction [2]. We have shown that, when expressed in Chinese hamster ovary cells, both WT and mutated GHRHR have a similar degree of expression proving that the missense mutations do not interfere with the posttranscriptional events. The mutant receptors display reduced ligand binding compared to the WT, impairing the receptor ability to transmit the intracellular signaling, in agreement with the idea that TM domains have a fundamental role in binding specificity [14].

GHRHR Polymorphisms

Several polymorphisms in the *GHRHR* have been reported, but their association with disease has not been fully elucidated yet. Recently, a study from a Swedish group reported two haplotypes for *GHRHR* account for as much as 1.8% of the variation in height after adjusting for age, sex and population affinity, making them the strongest contributor to normal variation in height identified so far [15].

GHRHR Involvement in Pituitary Adenoma Formation

Because elevated cAMP appears to be related to the excess somatotroph cell proliferation, it was logical to investigate the potential role of GHRHR alternative forms in causing somatotroph cell hyperplasia and adenoma formation [2]. Two studies have looked at the possible presence of somatic activating *GHRHR* mutations in GH-secreting adenomas, and neither found evidence for such mutations [16].

Diseases Associated with Inactivating *GHRHR* Mutations

Homozygous Phenotype

All the patients with biallelic mutations present a similar phenotype characterized by a severe degree of GH deficiency (GHD). Because GH and GHRH are not necessary during fetal life, children have normal size at birth, and the growth retardation becomes evident during the first year of age. Affected subjects show proportionate short stature, but not microphallus or dysmorphisms [17]. No case of neonatal hypoglycemia has been reported to date. Subjects respond well to GH replacement therapy (GHRT), with no evidence of slowing response that may indicate the development of anti-GH antibodies. Puberty usually occurs with delay in untreated subjects, without affecting fertility in either gender. GHD women from the Itabaianinha kindred tend to have a lower number of children possibly due to the delayed age of first intercourse and the necessity to perform caesarean section because of cephalic/pelvic disproportions. They have normal timing and symptoms of menopause. Despite a mild decrease in serum prolactin seen at age of climacteric, breastfeeding ability does not seem to be affected [2]. Adult height in untreated subjects is similar in the two largest kindreds described to date: 130.3 ± 10.6 cm in Sindh and 128.7 ± 5.9 in Itabaianinha for males, and 113.5 ± 0.7 cm in Sindh and 117.6 ± 5.7 cm in Itabaianinha for females. Height standard deviation decreases as child's age increases, reflecting the effects of cumulative GHD during life [6–7, 17].

Although different degrees of serum GH response to different stimuli have been reported (all of them well within the pathological level) due to different ethnic backgrounds, different ages at diagnosis, and multi-gene influence on stature, at present no obvious genotype-phenotype correlation can be drawn for individual mutations.

In the Itabaianinha IGHD subjects, serum concentrations of IGF-1, IGF-2, IGFBP3 and the acid-labile subunit are all markedly reduced, with complete separation from normal individuals at all ages of life. GHD is confirmed by the absent or markedly reduced responsiveness to any of the stimulation tests used (insulin, clonidine, GHRH and L-dopa), even when patients were pretreated with daily injections of GHRH for 6 days, confirming the complete resistance to GHRH [2]. A small but significant response to a GH secretagogue (GHRP-2), which acts on the ghrelin receptor, suggests a GHRH-independent effect of this substance on the somatotroph cells. Affected subjects have normal cortisol response to insulin-induced hypoglycemia [2].

Several studies have focused on pituitary MRI findings in these subjects. In agreement with the hypoplastic pituitary found in the *little* mouse, MRIs from adults and children of both Sindh and Itabaianinha kindreds show anterior pituitary hypoplasia (APH) in the majority of the cases. Because somatotroph cells account for 50–60% of pituitary cell mass, their lack of development in the absence of GHRH stimulus is the probable cause of APH, although pathology data from humans are not available. The physiological enlargement of the gland occurring in normal adolescents does not seem to occur in the affected subjects [12]. Although common, APH is not invariably present in patients with *GHRHR* mutations. It is not exclusive of them either. Whether APH is present at birth or develops during early childhood is not known. Recently, we reported a family with a *GHRHR* mutation in which two of the affected children had frank APH before age 6 [12].

The metabolic consequences of severe GHD are already present in early childhood. It is well known that GH has a direct lipolytic effect, and it increases hepatic gluconeogenesis and glycogenolysis. As expected, IGHD children and adolescents from the Itabaianinha kindred show high serum total and LDL cholesterol levels, decreased fat-free mass and increased percent fat mass, but only about 20% of them are overweight compared to the controls [18], and all the subjects have the expected initial lipolytic response to GHRT [2, 17].

Because the GH-IGF-1 axis plays an important role in bone metabolism and IGF-1 levels are correlated with bone mineral density, the bone status of the Itabaianinha GHD subjects was studied showing that adult subjects have reduced heel quantitative ultrasound T scores compared to controls, and that 6 months of depot GHRT induces a biochemical pattern of bone anabolism persisting for at least 6 months after the end of treatment [19].

GH and IGF-1 are also well known to affect myocardial contractility by increasing intracellular calcium and enhancing calcium sensitivity of myofilaments. To assess the impact of severe long-term IGHD on cardiac morphology and function, echocardiography was performed on 22 adult subjects from the Itabaianinha kindred [20]. Despite the higher prevalence of hypertension (commonly associated with increased left ventricular mass), GHD subjects do not show evidence of cardiac hypertrophy, suggesting that the very low IGF-1 levels might counterbalance the effects of the increased blood pressure. Conversely, GHRT causes an increase in all the parameters related to left ventricular mass [21].

Using ultrasonography to measure abdominal organ size, when corrected for body surface area, spleen and uterus show a relative reduction in volume, prostate and ovaries are proportionate to BSA, while pancreas, liver and kidney appear larger compared to the controls [17]. Reduction in spleen volume can be explained considering the important role of GH in hematolymphopoiesis, whereas the fact that women have a lower number of children might contribute to the reduced uterine size [22].

In addition, GHD individuals present a reduced thyroid volume associated with low serum T_3 and high serum free T_4 levels. This is probably due to the reduced trophic effect of IGF-1 on the thyrocytes and to the absence of GH stimulatory effect on peripheral T_4 to T_3 deiodination [2].

Affected subjects from both Sindh and Itabaianinha kindreds show a characteristic high-pitched voice, with the fundamental frequency (f0) similar in both males and females but higher than normal-height controls [23]. The high pitch is therefore particularly evident in males. GH might play the most relevant role in the development of voice quality mostly increasing vocal cord thickness. This particular rough and strained kind of voice, marked in males after puberty, derives in part from the size of their larynx and vocal cord length, but probably another important role is given by the reduced craniofacial dimensions with undeveloped nasopharyngeal cavities and abnormal pneumatized craniofacial bones [23].

Recently, we have reported that IGHD subjects from Itabaianinha have a higher prevalence of periodontal disease than local controls, possibly secondary to a lack of immunomodulatory effect of GH [24].

Due to previous studies showing increased vascular mortality in hypopituitary patients not treated with GHRT, a susceptibility to premature atherosclerosis has been hypothesized in untreated GHD subjects. Despite the evidence that lifelong IGHD is associated with several cardiovascular risk factors, such as central obesity, elevated blood pressure, and elevated serum cholesterol and C-reactive protein levels, it seems that acquired GHD has a more relevant impact on atherosclerosis than congenital GHD. In fact, GHD people from the Itabaianinha kindred do not show any evidence of premature atherosclerosis, or increase in carotid intima-media thickness [20]. This surprising findings could be attributed to the dual role of IGF-1 in atherosclerosis pathophysiology: it promotes atherogenesis by increasing vascular smooth muscle cell proliferation, but it also protects against it by increasing nitric oxide formation, vascular compliance and insulin sensitivity. Therefore, it has been suggested that a very low level of IGF-1 might have a protective role, whereas a milder decrease might be noxious. In addition, an increase in serum adiponectin and reduction in insulin resistance may explain such beneficial outcome. Interestingly, a 6-month treatment with depot GH, despite the modest increase in IGF-1 levels, improved lipid profile and body composition, but also increased significantly the carotid intima-media thickness and induced the development of carotid atherosclerotic plaques [21].

With regard to the influence of IGHD on longevity, the exact role of the GH-IGF-1 axis in humans is still controversial. Studies performed in several animal species show that the disruption of this axis increases life span [25]. In contrast, it is well known that GHD causes changes in body composition that are very similar to those occurring during aging. Since the previously reported epidemiological studies mostly included subjects with panhypopituitarism after surgery or radiation, it has been difficult to understand whether the increased cardiovascular mortality derived from untreated GHD or from these confounding factors. The Itabaianinha kindred represents a great opportunity to study GHD not associated with other diseases. Studies on this kindred suggest normal longevity of IGHD subjects. The only difference seems to be a higher frequency of early deaths in young IGHD females, which suggests a role of simultaneous lack of GH and estrogens. No differences have been found in the rate of cardiovascular deaths after adulthood is reached, despite the risk factors associated with GHD, or in the rate of cancer deaths [25]. These data are remarkably similar to what was recently reported by Guevara-Aguirre et al. [26], who studied an Ecuadorian cohort of 99 people with GH receptor deficiency (Laron's dwarfs) showing normal longevity and actually a lower incidence or delayed occurrence of neoplasms and diabetes.

Finally, IGHD people from Itabaianinha underwent a validated international questionnaire to assess quality of life (QoL) and, possibly because short stature is well accepted in this community, they showed no difference with the general population. Not surprisingly, GHRT does not improve QoL in these individuals. This observation, together with the detrimental effects on cardiovascular status, should be considered before starting GHRT in adults with previously untreated congenital GHD.

Heterozygous Phenotype

HTZ subjects from the Itabaianinha kindred show no significant difference in height compared to the non-mutation carriers from the same kindred. They have however lower fat-free mass, lower waist and hip circumference, and levels of insulin/HOMA-IR compatible with increased insulin sensitivity. It has been hypothesized that a small reduction in GH levels might cause these changes in body composition without affecting height. Even if these findings support the initial hypothesis of an intermediate phenotype in HTZ carriers, more studies are required to determine whether the HTZ status is associated with detectable reduction of GH secretion [27].

Conclusions

Due to their relatively high prevalence, *GHRHR* mutations should be suspected in children with early growth retardation due to IGHD, particularly in those patients with positive family history for growth failure and/or parental consanguinity. Although MRI evidence of APH should increase such suspicion, its absence does not exclude them. Unfortunately, despite the evidence of the important role played by *GHRHR* mutations in causing growth deficiency, no commercial screening is available to date, and their detection is limited to research laboratories. Nevertheless, genetic analysis is important for family counseling, and it is useful to predict both the phenotype and response to replacement therapy.

References

1 Alatzoglou KS, Alatzoglou KS, Turton JP, et al: Expanding the spectrum of mutations in GH1 and GHRHR: genetic screening in a large cohort of patients with congenital isolated growth hormone deficiency. J Clin Endocrinol Metab 2009;94:3191–3199.

2 Martari M, Salvatori R: Diseases associated with growth hormone-releasing hormone receptor (GHRHR) mutations. Prog Mol Biol Transl Sci 2009;88:57–84.

3 Mullis PE: Genetics of GHRH, GHRH-receptor, GH and GH-receptor: its impact on pharmacogenetics. Best Pract Res Clin Endocrinol Metab 2011;25:25–41.

4 Lin-Su K, Wajnrajch MP: Growth Hormone Releasing Hormone (GHRH) and the GHRH Receptor. Rev Endocr Metab Disord 2002;3:313–323.

5 Lam KS, Lee MF, Tam SP, Srivastava G: Gene expression of the receptor for growth-hormone-releasing hormone is physiologically regulated by glucocorticoids and estrogen. Neuroendocrinology 1996;63:475–480.

6 Salvatori R, Hayashida CY, Aguiar-Oliveira MH, Phillips JA 3rd, Souza AH, Gondo RG, Toledo SP, Conceicão MM, Prince M, Maheshwari HG, Baumann G, Levine MA: Familial dwarfism due to a novel mutation of the growth hormone-releasing hormone receptor gene. J Clin Endocrinol Metab 1999;84:917–923.

7 Maheshwari HG, Silverman BL, Dupuis J, Baumann G: Phenotype and genetic analysis of a syndrome caused by an inactivating mutation in the growth hormone-releasing hormone receptor: dwarfism of Sindh. J Clin Endocrinol Metab 1998;83:4065–4074.

8 Desai MP, Upadhye PS, Kamijo T, Yamamoto M, Ogawa M, Hayashi Y, Seo H, Nair SR: Growth hormone releasing hormone receptor (GHRH-r) gene mutation in Indian children with familial isolated growth hormone deficiency: a study from western India. J Pediatr Endocrinol Metab 2005;18:955–973.

9 Siklar Z, Berberoğlu M, Legendre M, Amselem S, Evliyaoğlu O, Hacıhamdioğlu B, Savaş Erdeve S, Oçal G: Two siblings with isolated GH deficiency due to loss-of-function mutation in the GHRHR gene: successful treatment with growth hormone despite late admission and severe growth retardation. J Clin Res Pediatr Endocrinol 2010;2:164–167.

10 Hilal L, Hajaji Y, Vie-Luton MP, Ajaltouni Z, Benazzouz B, Chana M, Chraïbi A, Kadiri A, Amselem S, Sobrier ML: Unusual phenotypic features in a patient with a novel splice mutation in the GHRHR gene. Mol Med 2008;14:286–292.

11 Salvatori R, Fan X, Phillips JA 3rd, Espigares-Martin R, Martin De Lara I, Freeman KL, Plotnick L, Al-Ashwal A, Levine MA: Three new mutations in the gene for the growth hormone (GH)-releasing hormone receptor in familial isolated GH deficiency type IB. J Clin Endocrinol Metab 2001;86:273–279.

12 Shohreh R, Sherafat-Kazemzadeh R, Jee YH, Blitz A, Salvatori R: A novel frame shift mutation in the GHRH receptor gene in familial isolated GH deficiency: early occurrence of anterior pituitary hypoplasia. J Clin Endocrinol Metab 2011;96:2982–2986.

13 Godi M, Mellone S, Petri A, Arrigo T, Bardelli C, Corrado L, Bellone S, Prodam F, Momigliano-Richiardi P, Bona G, Giordano M: A recurrent signal peptide mutation in the growth hormone releasing hormone receptor with defective translocation to the cell surface and isolated growth hormone deficiency. J Clin Endocrinol Metab 2009;94:3939–3947.

14 Alba M, Salvatori R: Naturally-occurring missense mutations in the human growth hormone-releasing hormone receptor alter ligand binding. J Endocrinol 2005;186:515–521.

15 Johansson A, Jonasson I, Gyllensten U: Extended haplotypes in the growth hormone releasing hormone receptor gene (GHRHR) are associated with normal variation in height. PLoS One 2009;4:e4464.

16 Salvatori R, Thakker RV, Lopes MB, Fan X, Eswara JR, Ellison D, Lees P, Harding B, Yang I, Levine MA: Absence of mutations in the growth hormone (GH)-releasing hormone receptor gene in GH-secreting pituitary adenomas. Clin Endocrinol (Oxf) 2001;54:301–307.

17 Aguiar Oliveira MH, Salvatori R: Lifetime growth hormone deficiency: impact on growth; in Preedy VR (ed): The Handbook of Growth and Growth Monitoring in Health and Disease. Berlin, Springer, 2011.

18 Gleeson H, Barreto ES, Salvatori R, Costa L, Oliveira CR, Pereira RM, Clayton P, Aguiar-Oliveira MH: Metabolic effects of growth hormone (GH) replacement in children and adolescents with severe isolated GH deficiency due to a GHRH receptor mutation. Clin Endocrinol (Oxf) 2007;66:466–474.

19 de Paula FJ, Góis-Júnior MB, Aguiar-Oliveira MH, Pereira Fde A, Oliveira CR, Pereira RM, Farias CT, Vicente TA, Salvatori R: Consequences of lifetime isolated growth hormone (GH) deficiency and effects of short-term GH treatment on bone in adults with a mutation in the GHRH-receptor gene. Clin Endocrinol (Oxf) 2009;70:35–40.

20 Menezes Oliveira JL, Marques-Santos C, Barreto-Filho JA, et al: Lack of evidence of premature atherosclerosis in untreated severe isolated growth hormone (GH) deficiency due to a GH-releasing hormone receptor mutation. J Clin Endocrinol Metab 2006;91:2093–2099.
21 Oliveira JL, Aguiar-Oliveira MH, D'Oliveira A Jr, et al: Congenital growth hormone (GH) deficiency and atherosclerosis: effects of GH replacement in GH-naive adults. J Clin Endocrinol Metab 2007;92: 4664–4670.
22 Oliveira CR, Salvatori R, Nóbrega LM, Carvalho EO, Menezes M, Farias CT, Britto AV, Pereira RM, Aguiar-Oliveira MH: Sizes of abdominal organs in adults with severe short stature due to severe, untreated, congenital GH deficiency caused by a homozygous mutation in the GHRH receptor gene. Clin Endocrinol (Oxf) 2008;69:153–158.
23 Barreto VM, D'Avila JS, Sales NJ, Gonçalves MI, Seabra JD, Salvatori R, Aguiar-Oliveira MH: Laryngeal and vocal evaluation in untreated growth hormone deficient adults. Otolaryngol Head Neck Surg 2009;140:37–42.
24 Britto IM, Aguiar-Oliveira MH, Oliveira-Neto LA, Salvatori R, Souza AH, Araujo VP, Corraini P, Pannuti CM, Romito GA, Pustiglioni FE: Periodontal disease in adults with untreated congenital growth hormone deficiency: a case-control study. J Clin Periodontol 2011;38:525–531.
25 Aguiar-Oliveira MH, Oliveira FT, Pereira RM, et al: Longevity in untreated congenital growth hormone deficiency due to a homozygous mutation in the GHRH receptor gene. J Clin Endocrinol Metab 2010;95:714–721.
26 Guevara-Aguirre J, Balasubramanian P, Guevara-Aguirre M, et al: Growth hormone receptor deficiency is associated with a major reduction in pro-aging signaling, cancer, and diabetes in humans. Sci Transl Med 2011;3:70ra13.
27 Pereira RM, Aguiar-Oliveira MH, Sagazio A, et al: Heterozygosity for a mutation in the growth hormone-releasing hormone receptor gene does not influence adult stature, but affects body composition. J Clin Endocrinol Metab 2007;92:2353–2357.

Roberto Salvatori, MD
Division of Endocrinology, Johns Hopkins University
1830 East Monument St. #333
Baltimore, MD 21287 (USA)
E-Mail salvator@jhmi.edu

Maghnie M, Loche S, Cappa M, Ghizzoni L, Lorini R (eds): Hormone Resistance and Hypersensitivity. From Genetics to Clinical Management. Endocr Dev. Basel, Karger, 2013, vol 24, pp 118–127 (DOI: 10.1159/000342586)

Current Issues on Molecular Diagnosis of GH Signaling Defects

Eva Feigerlova · Vivian Hwa · Michael A. Derr · Ron G. Rosenfeld

Department of Pediatrics, Oregon Health and Science University, Portland, Oreg., USA

Abstract

The growth-promoting effects of GH are mediated primarily by regulating the biosynthesis of insulin-like growth factor (IGF)-1. The binding of circulating GH to the cell surface GH receptor (GHR) initiates signaling cascades, of which the signal transducer and activator of transcription (STAT)-5b pathway has proven, in both rodent models and human case studies, to be the most critical in regulating IGF-1 production. The identification of rare inactivating *STAT5B* mutations in children, whose severe postnatal growth retardation was associated with GH insensitivity (GHI) and IGF-1 deficiency, confirmed the importance of STAT5b in regulating IGF-1 gene expression. Unlike GHI due to mutations in the *GHR* gene, patients carrying *STAT5B* mutations often present with immune dysfunction that can lead to severe, life-threatening infections and chronic pulmonary disease, consistent with the fact that STAT5b is activated by multiple cytokines involved in immunity. The possibility of a STAT5b disorder should be considered, therefore, when children present with chronic infection and/or unexplained pulmonary disease concomitant with severe postnatal growth failure.

The growth-promoting effects of pituitary-derived GH are mediated largely, if not exclusively, by insulin-like growth factor 1 (IGF-1), both circulating and locally produced. GH regulates IGF-1 production via activation of the GH receptor (GHR) signaling system. Upon binding to GH, the homodimeric GHR, which lacks intrinsic kinase activity, recruits cytosolic Janus kinase 2 (JAK2) and, subsequently, activates multiple signaling pathways, including the signal transducer and activator of transcription (STAT)-1, -3, -5a, -5b, pathways, the MAPK (mitogen-activated protein kinase) and the PI3K (phosphoinositide-3 kinase) pathways, culminating in the regulation of multiple genes, including *IGF1* (fig. 1). GH-regulated IGF-I circulates in serum as a ternary complex with the IGF-binding protein (IGFBP)-3 and acid labile subunit (ALS), both of which are also regulated by the GH-GHR system. The critical importance of the GHR-JAK2-STAT5b pathway for IGF-1 production and normal postnatal growth in humans has been demonstrated by analysis of patients with

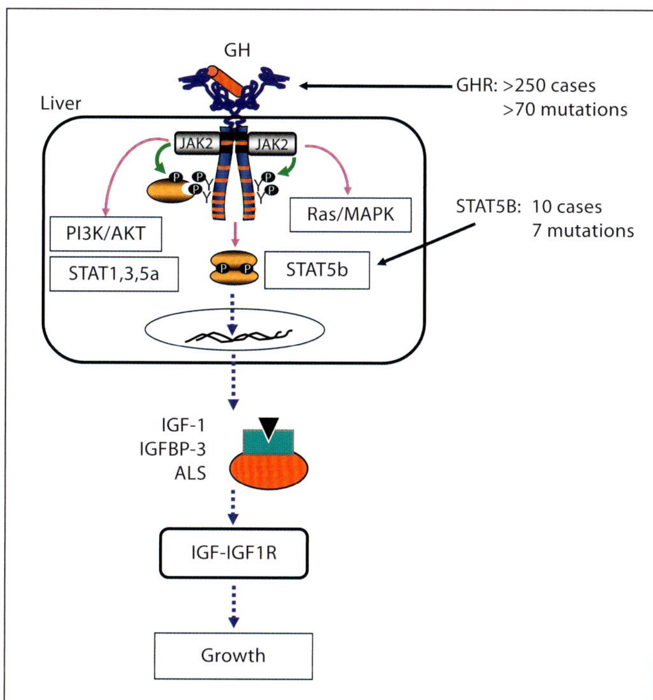

Fig. 1. The GH-IGF-1 axis. Signaling pathways induced upon binding of GH to homodimeric GHR and JAK2-mediated phosphorylation (P) of tyrosines (Y) in the intracellular domain of GHR are indicated. The signaling pathway is discussed in the text.

GH insensitivity (GHI), which is defined by normal or elevated basal and stimulated serum GH associated with low serum IGF-1 and a lack of response to exogenous GH therapy [1]. The earliest identified cases of severe GHI were found to be the result of mutations of *GHR*. Subsequently, however, cases of severe growth failure, GHI and IGF-1 deficiency (IGFD) were identified in patients with normal *GHR*, but associated with mutations of the *STAT5B* gene [2, 3]. These cases constituted the first demonstration, in humans, that the STAT5b signaling pathway is critical for both IGF-1 production and normal growth.

GHR-IGF-1 Axis: STAT5b Pathway

The GHR, a homodimeric transmembrane protein, binds circulating GH, and this GH-GHR interaction induces signal transduction through recruitment and activation of the cytosolic JAK2. Activated JAK2 subsequently phosphorylates both itself and tyrosine residues in the cytoplasmic domain of GHR. Recently, it has been demonstrated that 3 intracellular tyrosines of the human GHR (Y534, Y566 or Y627) are critical and redundant in the GH-induced STAT5b signaling process [4]. The phosphorylated tyrosines act as docking sites for signaling components, such as STAT5b. JAK2 phosphorylates the docked STAT5b on a single tyrosine (Tyr699) (fig. 2), and the

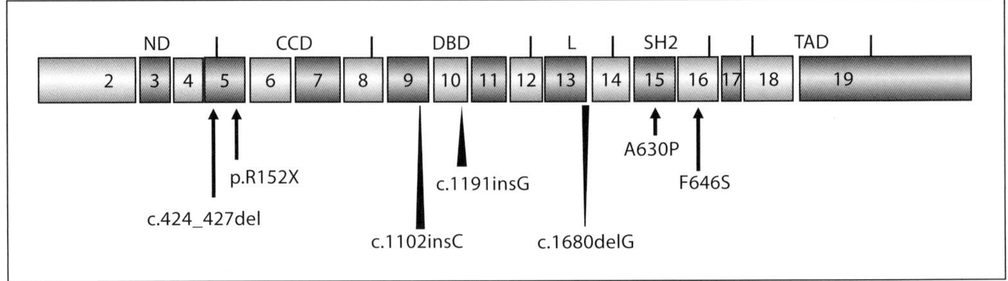

Fig. 2. Schematic representation of protein domains in the human STAT5b protein. Tyrosine 699 (Y699) that is phosphorylated by JAK2 is shown. Mutations identified are indicated.

phosphorylated STAT5b subsequently dissociates from the GHR and forms homodimers. Homodimeric phospho-STAT5b translocates to the nucleus, where it binds DNA and regulates gene transcription, including the *IGF1* gene (fig. 1). In rodent models, recent reports suggested that GH-stimulated phospho-Stat5b associated with multiple dispersed DNA segments, i.e. GH response elements (GHRE), within the *Igf1* locus for induction of *Igf1* gene transcription [5, 6]. In contrast, GHREs within the human *IGF1* locus have yet to be identified, but may be analogous to rat *Igf1* GHRE. Interestingly, there is no evidence to date that in humans, the very closely related STAT5a (>90% similarity with STAT5b) is involved in GH-induced production of IGF-1.

Current Status of GH Signaling Defects

The biological effects of GH can only be obtained in the presence of a normal functioning GHR and an intact postreceptor signaling pathway. Over 70 GHR mutations have been identified in more than 250 clinical cases of GHI, and are mainly associated with structural abnormalities of the GHR extracellular domain [1, 7]. The majority of *GHR* mutations are recessive, with only three dominant negative heterozygous GHR mutations described to date [8–10]. The first report of a specific molecular defect in GH signal transduction was published by Kofoed et al. [2] in 2003. Currently, seven unique *STAT5B* mutations have been identified in 10 reported STAT5b-deficient patients [3, 7] (table 1).

STAT5b Is the Critical Mediator of GH-Induced IGF-1 Production

The STAT5b protein is a member of the STAT family of transcription factors (STAT1, -2, -3, -4, -5a, -5b, and -6) that are activated by hormones (e.g. GH and prolactin) and cytokines (e.g. interferon-γ, IL-2, and IL-7). STATs 1, 3, 5a and 5b are recruited to the cytoplasmic domain of the GHR. The binding of STAT5b (and STAT5a) via its SH2 domain (see below), to key GHR cytoplasmic phosphorylated tyrosines allows STAT5b to be phosphorylated by activated JAK2 [4]. In contrast, GH activation of STAT3 and STAT1 does not require docking to phosphotyrosines on GHR, supporting the concept that GH is capable of activating STAT signaling pathways by more than one mechanism [4, 11]. Of these STAT pathways, recent studies show, the STAT5b pathway is the principal, if not the sole, signaling pathway in humans for GH-induced, IGF-1-mediated postnatal growth. The first evidence for this was provided through murine models involving inactivation of the STAT5a or STAT5b genes. Animals presented with severe growth impairment, low serum IGF-1 levels and the absence of IGF-1 expression in response to exogenous GH [12–15]. In these rodent models, unlike in humans, both STAT5a and -5b appeared to be involved in GH-induced IGF-1 production.

Inactivating mutations in the *STAT5B* gene have been described in 10 patients with severe growth retardation, thus confirming the key role of STAT5b in GH-mediated IGF-1 production [2, 3]. From the perspective of auxology, phenotypes of these patients were similar to those of patients with mutations in the GHR gene, indicating that the presence of normal STAT5a could not compensate for lost STA5b function. STAT5a and STAT5b, thus, do not appear to be fully redundant in humans [16]. Unlike the murine models, where a sexual dimorphism of the STAT5b function was observed, with only affected males being growth retarded [12, 13], 7 of the 10 reported patients were females. This finding indicates that in humans, STAT5b plays an essential role in the growth of both sexes, consistent with the observation of relatively little dimorphism in stature (especially prepubertally) in humans. These observations do not exclude the possibility that GH-IGF-1 signaling may be modulated by additional physiological and pathological events which might influence IGF-1 gene regulation, however. Recently, a possibly broader role for Stat5b in controlling IGF-1 gene expression via other non-GH-activated regulatory pathways has been proposed [6].

STAT5b Protein and Molecular Defects Identified in Humans

The human STAT5b gene, located on chromosome 17q11.2, contains 19 exons, encoding a protein of 787 amino acids that consists of several domains (fig. 2). Each domain carries specific function(s): the N-terminal domain (ND) and the coiled-coiled domain participate in protein-protein interactions; the DNA-binding domain (DBD); the linker region (L) whose function(s) is unclear; the highly conserved modular SH2 domain allows STAT proteins to bind phosphorylated tyrosines, and the C-terminal transactivation domain is important for interacting with other transcriptional factors.

Since the first report of a patient carrying a homozygous missense mutation, p.Ala630Pro (p.A630P), in the SH2 domain of the STAT5B gene [2], only 9 other

Table 1. Phenotype of patients with STAT5b deficiency

	Kofoed	Hwa	Bercasconi	Boyanovsky
	[2]	[19]	[24]	[25]
Observation				
Consanguinity	yes	yes	ND	adopted
Paternal height SDS	–0.3	–0.9	–2.2	NA
Mother height SDS	–1.2	–0.6	–3.3	NA
Sex of proband	F	F	F	F
Age years	16.5	16.4	15.3	12
Height SDS	–7.5	–7.8	–9.9	–5.3
Puberty	delayed	delayed	delayed	delayed
CPD	yes	yes	yes	yes
Atopy	eczema	eczema	eczema	eczema
Other		bleeding diathesis		thyroiditis
Hormonal evaluation				
GH basal ng/ml	9.4	14.2	6.6	1.8
GH stimulated ng/ml	53.8 (H)	NA	NA	12.5
IGF-1 ng/ml[1]	38	7.0	< 10	0.8
IGF-1, GH stimulated ng/ml[2]	55	NA	NA	0.8
IGFBP-3 mg/l[1]	0.87	0.54	NA	0.5
ALS mg/l[1]	2.9	1.2	NA	0.7
Prolactin	102-168 (H)	NA	169 (H)	13–15
Molecular defect	p.A630P	*c.1191insG*	p.R152X	p.R152X

Homozygous *STAT5B* mutations were identified in 10 case reports (modified [7]). Birthweight and length (not shown) were normal for gestation. Height SDS (of probands) is at first observation or as reported. Molecular defects encompass missense and non-sense mutations (nomenclature, protein designation), and frameshifts due to insertion or deletion of exonic nucleotides (nomenclature, in italics, based on cDNA). JIA = Juvenile idiopathic arthritis; NA = not available; CPD = chronic pulmonary disease; H = high, above normal of 20 µg/l. [1] All reported values are significantly below the normal range (methodology varied from site to site). [2] Value determined after 7 days of daily GH injections (at 50 µg/kg bodyweight).

STAT5b-deficient patients have been described [3, 17]. One patient carried a missense mutation, also in the SH2 domain [17], while the remaining patients carried non-sense or frameshift mutations within the *STAT5B* gene. The STAT5b mutations described in all cases to date are autosomal recessive.

The first described STAT5b mutation, the A630P substitution, disrupted the core of anti-parallel β-sheets that forms the phosphate-binding pocket, causing reduced thermodynamic stability, aberrant folding and diminished solubility of the mutant STAT5b protein [18]. We recently provided functional analysis of the second missense STAT5B mutations (p.F646S) compared to p.A630P, both localized in the SH2

Vidarsdottir	Hwa [20]		Publiese-Pires [21]		Scaglia
[22]	sibling 1	sibling 2	sibling 1	sibling 2	[17]
ND	yes	yes	ND	ND	adopted
–0.8	–1.28	–1.28	–1.5	–1.5	NA
–2.8	–0.6	–0.6	–1.0	–1.0	NA
M	F	F	M	M	F
31	2	4	6	2	19
–5.9	–5.8	–5.6	–5.6	–3	–5.90
delayed	NA	NA	delayed	NA	normal
no	yes	yes	yes	yes	no
ichthyosis			atopic	atopic	eczema
Sickle cell anemia	JIA			thrombocytopenic purpura	thyroiditis
0.13	17.7	5.7	1.7	1	NA
14.2	NA	NA	20.6	14	27.1
8	<5	<5	34	<25	16
NA	NA	NA	48	<25	12
0.18	0.7	0.8	0.52	0.75	0.84
0.7	0.4	0.8	NA	NA	NA
110 (H)	NA	NA	61.1 (H)	76.6 (H)	83 (H)
c.1102insC	*c.1680delG*	*c.1680delG*	*c.424_427del*	*c.424_427del*	p.F646S

domain [17]. Reconstitution studies have demonstrated a lack of transcriptional activities of the p.F646S mutation, despite GH-induced phosphorylation, and provided further evidence for the importance of the SH2 domain for full STAT5b transcriptional activities [17].

Of the five other unique *STAT5B* mutations described to date (fig. 2), one nonsense and four frameshift *STAT5B* mutations, none to date has been experimentally evaluated for expression and biological actions, but each would be predicted to lead to nonfunctional STAT5b proteins.

Clinical and Biochemical Features of STAT5b Deficiency

Growth and Puberty

Intrauterine growth and birth parameters in STAT5b-deficient subjects are within the normal range. Severe postnatal growth failure is observed, however, with height SDS ranging from –3.0 to –9.9 SDS in both sexes [3]. Modestly delayed puberty was noted in subjects for whom data were available. Mild facial dysmorphic features, such as a prominent forehead, depressed nasal bridge and high-pitched voice, were noted for some of the STAT5b deficient subjects, similar to that observed with *GHR* mutations.

Limited data are currently available concerning the phenotype of the heterozygote state, although observations suggest a modest degree of growth failure (SDS ranging from –0.3 to –3.3) [3].

Biochemical Features

GH levels at baseline were found to be normal to elevated, with normal GHBP values, and severe deficiencies of IGF-1, IGFBP-3, and ALS. These patients do not respond to either endogenous or exogenous GH in terms of growth, metabolic changes or significant elevations of serum concentrations of the GH-dependent growth factors IGF-1, IGFBP-3 or ALS. It is of note that elevated prolactin levels were observed in those patients with recorded concentrations.

Effects on Immunity

STAT5b deficiency has been associated with immune dysregulation [3]. Clinical symptoms presented by the patients include severe infections, lymphocytic interstitial pneumonitis, juvenile idiopathic arthritis, thrombocytopenic purpura, and autoimmune thyroiditis [17, 19–21]. Two of the patients died as consequences of progressive pulmonary fibrosis and respiratory failure, and one underwent successful lung transplantation at age 17.5 years [3, 21].

The immunological profile of the STAT5b-deficient patients showed decreased numbers of regulatory CD4+CD25^{high} T cells (T reg), low levels of CD8, low NK activity, and elevated activated CD4^{+}CD45RO^{+} [3, 17]. These findings suggested the importance of STAT5b proteins in immune homeostasis and regulation of cytokine systems. It is of note that in the reported STAT5b-deficient cases, only one was not severely immunocompromised and had a normal immune profile, despite carrying a homozygous nucleotide insertion in the DNA-binding domain [22, 23].

Recommendations

The 10 cases of homozygous *STAT5b* mutations identified to date have all presented with severe growth failure. Given the significance of the immunological dysregulation in 9/10 of these patients, it appears likely that some cases currently followed in immunology and pulmonary clinics may have undiagnosed underlying STAT5b defects. A STAT5b disorder should be suspected in children with chronic infection and/or unexplained pulmonary disease concomitant with severe growth failure. In those children where presentation includes T cell lymphopenia and low concentrations of CD4+CD25^{high}, analysis of the STAT5b gene should be considered. Chronic lung disease in these patients can be severe and often leads to high morbidity and mortality; it is likely, therefore, that early diagnosis, regular monitoring and prophylactic therapy could improve the clinical outcomes for these subjects. Any symptoms of immunodeficiency should be treated with antimicrobial and/or immunosuppressive therapies for exaggerated effector T cell responses.

To manage growth failure in these patients, GH therapy is ineffective. IGF-1 therapy might represent a treatment option, providing that chronic infection is effectively controlled.

Conclusion

Our molecular understanding of GH-induced signal transduction has improved significantly over the past decades, and ongoing research provides us with valuable insights into the regulation of GH-IGF-1 signaling. The GHR-JAK2-STAT5b-IGF pathway is, at least in humans, the major endocrine mediator of growth.

The identification of rare *STAT5B* mutations has highlighted the distinct and critical role of STAT5b in both growth and immunity. The possibility of a STAT5b disorder in children should be considered by the general pediatrician when chronic infection and/or unexplained pulmonary disease are concomitant with growth failure.

Further research is needed to better understand genotype-phenotype correlations of STAT5b mutations, and to determine if heterozygous mutations are associated with a significant phenotype.

References

1 Savage MO, Attie KM, David A, Metherell LA, Clark AJ, Camacho-Hübner C: Endocrine assessment, molecular characterization and treatment of growth hormone insensitivity disorders. Nat Clin Pract Endocrinol Metab 2006;2:395–407.

2 Kofoed EM, Hwa V, Little B, Woods KA, Buckway CK, Tsubaki J, Pratt KL, Bezrodnik L, Jasper H, Tepper A, Heinrich J, Rosenfeld RG: Growth-hormone insensitivity (GHI) associated with a STAT-5b mutation. N Engl J Med 2003;349:1139–1147.

3 Hwa V, Nadeau K, Wit JM, Rosenfeld RG: STAT5b deficiency: lessons from STAT5b gene mutations. Best Pract Res Clin Endocrinol Metab 2011;25: 61–75.

4 Derr MA, Fang P, Sinha SK, Ten S, Hwa V, Rosenfeld RG: A novel Y332C missense mutation in the intracellular domain of the human growth hormone receptor does not alter STAT5b signaling: redundancy of GHR intracellular tyrosines involved in STAT5b signaling. Horm Res Paediatr 2011;75: 187–199.

5 Chia D, Varco-Merth B, Rotwein P: Dispersed chromosomal Stat5b-binding elements mediate growth hormone-activated insulin-like growth factor-I gene transcription. J Biol Chem 2010;285:17636–17647.

6 Rotwein P: Mapping the growth hormone-Stat5b-IGF-I transcriptional circuit. Trends Endocrinol Metab 2012;23:186–193.

7 David A, Hwa V, Metherell LA, Netchine I, Camacho-Hubner C, Clark AJ, Rosenfeld RG, Savage MO: Evidence for a continuum of genetic, phenotypic, and biochemical abnormalities in children with growth hormone insensitivity. Endo Rev 2011; 32:472–497.

8 Ayling RM, Ross R, Towner P, Von Laue S, Finidori J, Moutoussamy S, Buchanan CR, Clayton PE, Norman MR: A dominant negative mutation of the growth hormone receptor causes familial short stature. Nat Genet 1997;16:13–14.

9 Iida K, Takahashi Y, Kaji H, Nose O, Okimura Y, Abe H, Chihara K: Growth hormone (GH) insensitivity syndrome with high serum GH-binding protein levels caused by a heterozygous splice site mutation of the GH receptor gene producing a lack of intracellular domain. J Clin Endocrinol Metab 1998;83:531–537.

10 Derr MA, Aisenberg J, Fang P, Tenenbaum-Rakover Y, Rosenfeld RG, Hwa V: The growth hormone receptor (GHR) c.899dupC mutation functions as a dominant negative: insights into the pathophysiology of intracellular GHR defects. J Clin Endocrinol Metab 2011;96:1896–1904.

11 Milward A, Metherell L, Maamra M, Barahona MJ, Wilkinson IR, Camacho-Hubner C, Savage MO, Bidlingmaier CM, Clark AJL, Ross RJM, Webb SM: Growth hormone (GH) insensitivity syndrome due to a GH receptor truncated after Box1, resulting in isolated failure of STAT5 signal transduction. J Clin Endocrinol Metab 2004;89:1259–1266.

12 Liu X, Robinson GW, Wagner KU, Garrett L, Wynshaw-Boris A, Hennighausen L: Stat5a is mandatory for adult mammary gland development and lactogenesis. Genes Dev 1997;11:179–186.

13 Udy GB, Towers RP, Snell RG, Wilkins RJ, Park SH, Ram PA, Waxman DJ, Davey HW: Requirement of STAT5b for sexual dimorphism of body growth rates and liver gene expression. Proc Natl Acad Sci USA 1997;94:7239–7244.

14 Teglund S, McKay C, Schuetz E, van Deursen JM, Stravopodis D, Wang D, Brown M, Bodner S, Grosveld G, Ihle JN: Stat5a and Stat5b proteins have essential and nonessential, or redundant, roles in cytokine responses. Cell 1998;93:841–850.

15 Davey HW, Xie T, McLachian MJ, Wilkins RJ, Waxman DJ, Grattan DR: STAT5b is required for GH-induced liver IGF-I gene expression. Endocrinology 2001;142:3836–3841.

16 Hwa V, Little B, Kofoed EM, Rosenfeld RG: Transcriptional regulation of insulin-like growth factor-I (IGF-I) by interferon-gamma (INF-γ) requires Stat-5b. J Biol Chem 2004;279:2728–2231.

17 Scaglia PA, Martínez AS, Feigerlová E, Bezrodnik L, Gaillard MI, Di Giovanni D, Ballerini MG, Jasper HG, Heinrich JJ, Fang P, Domené HM, Rosenfeld RG, Hwa V: A novel missense mutation in the SH2 domain of the STAT5B gene results in a transcriptionally inactive STAT5b associated with severe IGF-I deficiency, immune dysfunction, and lack of pulmonary disease. J Clin Endocrinol Metab 2012; 97:E830–E839.

18 Chia DJ, Subbian E, Buck TM, Hwa V, Rosenfeld RG, Skach WR, Shinde U, Rotwein P: Aberrant folding of a mutant STAT5b causes growth hormone insensitivity and proteasomal dysfunction. J Biol Chem 2006;281:6552–6558.

19 Hwa V, Little B, Adiyaman P, Kofoed EM, Pratt KL, Ocal G, Berberoglu M, Rosenfeld RG: Severe growth hormone insensitivity resulting from total absence of signal transducer and activator of transcription 5b. J Clin Endocrinol Metab 2005;90: 4260–4266.

20 Hwa V, Camacho-Hubner C, Little BM, David A, Metherell LA, El-Khatib N, Savage MO, Rosenfeld RG: Growth hormone insensitivity and severe short stature in siblings: a novel mutation at the exon13-intron 13 junction of the STAT5b gene. Horm Res 2007;68:218–224.
21 Pugliese-Pires PN, Tonelli CA, Dora JM, Silva PC, Czepielewski M, Simoni G, Arnhold IJ, Jorge AA: A novel STAT5B mutation causing GH insensitivity syndrome associated with hyperprolactinemia and immune dysfunction in two male siblings. Eur J Endocrinol 2010;163:349–355.
22 Vidarsdottir S, Walenkamp MJE, Pereira AM, Karperien M, van Doorn J, van Duyvenvoorde HA, White S, Breuning MH, Roelfsema F, Femke Kruithof M, van Dissel J, Janssen R, Wit JM, Romijn JA: Clinical and biochemical characteristics of a male patient with a novel homozygous STAT5b mutation. J Clin Endocrinol Metab 2006;91:3482–3485.
23 Walenkamp MJ, Vidarsdottir S, Pereira AM, Karperien M, van Doorn J, van Duyvenvoorde HA, Breuning MH, Roelfsema F, Kruithof MF, van Dissel J, Janssen R, Wit JM, Romijn JA: Growth hormone secretion and immunological function of a male patient with a homozygous STAT5b mutation. Eur J Endocrinol 2007;156:155–165.
24 Bernasconi A, Marino R, Ribas A, Rossi J, Ciaccio M, Oleastro M, Ornani A, Paz R, Rivarola M, Zelazko M, Belgorosky A: Characterization of immunodeficiency in a patient with growth hormone insensitivity secondary to a novel STAT5b gene mutation. Pediatrics 2006;118:e1584–e1592.
25 Boyanovsky A, Lozano A, Testa G, Munoz L, Marino R, Bernasconi A, Belgorosky A, Miras M: Growth hormone insensitivity and immunodeficiency: mutation in the STAT5B gene; in 8th Joint Meet Lawson Wilkins Pediatr Endocr Soc/Eur Soc Paediatr Endocrinol, New York, September 2009, P01–P067.

Ron G. Rosenfeld
PO Box 1746
Los Altos, CA 04023 (USA)
E-Mail stat5consulting@yahoo.com

Maghnie M, Loche S, Cappa M, Ghizzoni L, Lorini R (eds): Hormone Resistance and Hypersensitivity. From Genetics to Clinical Management. Endocr Dev. Basel, Karger, 2013, vol 24, pp 128–137 (DOI: 10.1159/000342841)

Molecular IGF-1 and IGF-1 Receptor Defects: From Genetics to Clinical Management

M.J.E. Walenkamp[a] · M. Losekoot[b] · J.M. Wit[c]

[a]Department of Pediatrics, VU University Medical Center, Amsterdam, [b]Laboratory of Diagnostic Genome Analysis, Department of Clinical Genetics, and [c]Department of Pediatrics, Leiden University Medical Center, Leiden, The Netherlands

Abstract

Molecular defects of the insulin-like growth factor 1 gene *(IGF1)* are rare in the human. Only three homozygous and two families with heterozygous mutations of the *IGF1* gene have been described, resulting in a variable degree of intrauterine and postnatal growth retardation, microcephaly, developmental delay and deafness. Detailed genetic analysis and functional experiments have shown that IGF-1 plays a key role in pre- and postnatal growth and development in human. Eleven patients with heterozygous and 2 patients with compound heterozygous mutations in the type 1 IGF1 receptor gene *(IGF1R)* have been reported. Intrauterine and postnatal growth retardation, microcephaly and IGF-1 levels above the mean of age references are consistent findings in these patients, although IGF-1 levels can be low initially because of feeding problems. The first reported patients showed the most severe phenotype, but with the identification of additional patients the phenotype appears to be more variable. The functional effect of the defects has been studied by in vitro experiments. From these studies, receptor haploinsufficiency, decreased *IGF1R* biosynthesis, interference with ligand binding and transmembrane signaling, and disruption of the intrinsic tyrosine kinase activity have been suggested as possible mechanisms with a variable pathogenetic spectrum. Data on GH treatment in these children are limited, showing a poor to modest growth response.

Observations in animal models have shown that insulin-like growth factor 1 (IGF-1) plays a key role in intrauterine growth and development [1]. *IGF1* null mice are 65% of normal weight at birth, and most die shortly after birth, indicating that before birth IGF-1 is the major determinant of growth and development. These findings were in contrast to the normal birth size of severely growth hormone (GH)-deficient mice, suggesting that prenatal IGF-1 secretion is independent of GH [2]. Postnatal growth in GH-deficient mice is retarded, confirming the increasing role of GH in postnatal growth. Since the first report of a patient with a deletion of exon 4 and 5 of *IGF1* in 1996 [3], only 3 other patients with a homozygous *IGF1* mutation and two families

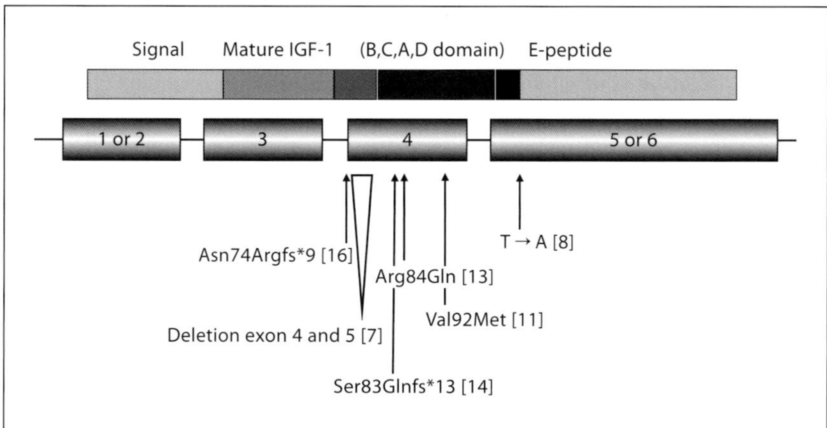

Fig. 1. Pre-pro IGF-1 protein with B, C, A and D domain of the mature protein and the exons of *IGF1* with homozygous (bold) and heterozygous mutations. T→A was described as a pathogenic mutation [8]; however, later this variant was found in normal-stature controls [10]. Val92Met was published as V44M [11] according to HGVS nomenclature Val92Met. Arg84Gln was published as R36Q [13], according to HGVS nomenclature Arg84Gln.

with heterozygous mutations of *IGF1* have been described. In this article, we review the molecular defects in these patients and their phenotype.

The metabolic effects of IGF-1 are mediated through the type 1 IGF-1 receptor (IGF1R). *IGF1R* null mice weigh 55% of wild-type littermates at birth, and die within a few hours after birth because of respiratory failure, showing organ hypoplasia, lung, skin, bone, and neurologic defects. Heterozygous *IGF1R*$^{+/-}$ mice were phenotypically normal, suggesting that a single functional *IGF1R* allele is sufficient to assure normal growth [4]. However, later experiments showed that targeted disruption of *IGF1R* (41% reduced availability) resulted in a growth deficit of 13% in male and 6% in female mice [5]. This suggests that a partial reduction in IGF-1 signaling reduces postnatal growth potential. Since the first report of 2 patients with a heterozygous *IGF1R* mutation in 2003 [6], many additional patients with heterozygous *IGF1R* defects have been identified. The variability of the phenotype and the molecular mechanisms will be reviewed.

Molecular *IGF1* Defects

IGF1 is located on the long arm of chromosome 12 (12q23.2). The mature IGF-1 peptide is a single-chain 70-amino acid protein encoded by exon 3 and 4, containing 4 domains (B, C, A, and D). The signal peptide encoded by exon 1 and 2, and the E-peptide encoded by exon 5 and/or 6 are posttranslationally removed (fig. 1). Besides the growth-promoting effect, IGF-1 has metabolic and mitogenic effects.

Table 1. Birth size, height and head circumference in patients with a homozygous *IGF1* defect

	Woods et al. [3]	Bonapace et al. [8]	Walenkamp et al. [25]	Netchine et al. [32]
Birthweight SDS	–3.9	–4.0	–3.9	–2.4
Birth length SDS	–5.4	–6.5	–4.3	–3.7
Head circ. at birth SDS	–4.9	–7.5		–2.5
Height SDS	–6.9	–6.1	–8.5	–4.9
Head circ. SDS	–5.3	–7.5	–8.0	–4.0

The first homozygous defect of the *IGF1* gene was described by Woods et al. [3] in 1996. Analysis of *IGF1* showed a homozygous deletion of exons 4 and 5 that is predicted to result in a mature IGF-1 peptide truncated from 70 to 25 amino acids. The phenotype of this patient consisted of severe intrauterine growth retardation (table 1), microcephaly, postnatal growth failure, severe psychomotor retardation, sensorineural deafness and mild dysmorphic features (micrognathia, ptosis and a low hairline). Biochemically IGF-1 levels were undetectable, even after GH stimulation. Spontaneous GH secretion was elevated. He was treated with rhIGF-1 at the age of 16.2 years, which increased his linear growth and insulin sensitivity [7]. His consanguineous parents and a sister were heterozygous for the defect. They had heights within the lower half of the normal range (father –1.8 SDS, mother –1.4 SDS, sister at 10 years –1 SDS).

In 2003, a patient with a similar clinical phenotype was described with extremely low serum levels of IGF-1 [8]. The authors found a homozygous T→A transversion in the untranslated region of exon 6 of *IGF1*, resulting in an altered E domain of the IGF-1 precursor. Treatment with rhIGF-1 for 7.5 years resulted in increased growth, and head circumference increased from –7.5 to –4.3 SDS [9]. However, in a later study, Coutinho et al. [10] identified this variant in a homozygous (n = 4) and heterozygous (n = 6) state in controls with a normal height varying from –0.1 to +2.4 SDS, indicating that this polymorphism does not cause IGF-1 deficiency and that the phenotype is possibly caused by a promotor or intronic defect.

In 2005, we described a patient with a homozygous missense mutation of *IGF1*. A homozygous G>A substitution at position 274 resulted in a substitution of a valine in domain A of the mature protein to a methionine at position 92, according to the Human Genome Variation Society (HGVS) nomenclature (published as position 44) [11]. Functional experiments showed a 90-fold lower binding affinity for the IGF1R due to subtle changes in the overall structure of the mutated protein [12]. As a consequence, phosphorylation of the IGF1R and downstream signaling proteins was diminished. Phenotypical features consisted of severe intrauterine growth retardation, postnatal growth retardation, microcephaly, severe mental retardation, sensorineural deafness and mild dysmorphic features including micrognathia. Serum IGF-1

Table 2. Auxological data and IGF-1 level of patients with heterozygous *IGF1R* defects [6, 18–25, 27, 29]

Birthweight SDS	−1.5 to −3.5
Birth length SDS	−0.3 to −5.0
Head circ. at birth SDS	−2.3 to −5.7
Height SDS	−2.1 to −7.3
IGF-1 SDS	> −0.6

was markedly elevated (+7.3 SDS), and stimulated GH secretion was in the upper normal range. We had the opportunity to investigate 9 heterozygous family members and 15 noncarriers. The heterozygous carriers had a lower birthweight (3,048 vs. 3,358 g), height (−1.0 vs. −0.4 SDS) and head circumference (−1.0 vs. 0.5 SDS) than the noncarriers, indicating a gene-dose effect on growth.

The most recently reported homozygous defect of *IGF1* showed a milder phenotype in a boy with moderate intrauterine growth retardation, normal hearing and mild developmental delay [13]. IGF-1 levels varied from undetectable to > +2 SDS according to the immunoassay used. GH secretion was slightly elevated. Treatment with high doses of GH (0.4 mg/kg/week) resulted in catch-up growth. Because of the normal IGFBP-3 levels, an *IGF1* defect was suspected and sequencing revealed a homozygous missense mutation replacing an arginine in position 84 (HGVS nomenclature, published as position 36) of the C domain by a glutamine. The mutant protein had a moderately lower affinity for the receptor (3.9 times) than the wild-type protein and was less effective in phosphorylating the receptor. This patient showed that the phenotype of a homozygous *IGF1* defect can be milder than the first patients suggested and that a patient with intrauterine and postnatal growth retardation, and microcephaly with abnormally low or high IGF-1 levels but normal IGFBP-3 warrant mutation analysis of *IGF1*.

While the heterozygous relatives of the homozygous index patients only showed a moderate effect on growth and head circumference, recently two families with severe short stature associated with a heterozygous *IGF1* defect have been described. Van Duyvenvoorde et al. [14] reported a heterozygous duplication of four nucleotides, resulting in a frameshift at position 83 of the mature IGF-1 protein and a premature stop codon in 4 family members. Carriers of the *IGF1* mutation tended to have a lower height SDS (−3.4 vs. −1.6) and had a significantly lower head circumference (−1.9 vs. 0.3). Tone audiometry was normal. Since the mutant protein is not able to bind to the IGF1R, the authors speculate that *IGF1* haploinsufficiency causes the growth retardation. Apparently, in this family one wild-type copy of *IGF1* cannot express sufficient IGF-1 (serum IGF-1 levels varied between −1.8 and −2.6 SDS). Interestingly, the probands who inherited the mutation from their mother showed a more severe phenotype than the mother, who inherited the mutation from her father. This suggests that maternal IGF-1 deficiency during pregnancy leads to placental dysfunction, affecting intrauterine growth. This is supported by studies showing a strong correlation between the rate of maternal IGF-1 increase during pregnancy [15].

Recently, a large kindred with severe short stature was reported, in which a heterozygous mutation of the *IGF1* gene was found to segregate with short stature [16]. Five relatives in 3 generations carried the mutation. Their height varied between –2.8 and –6.4 SDS, and no intrauterine growth retardation, microcephaly or deafness occurred. The mutation was located in intron 4, at the first invariant dinucleotide of the intron 4 donor splice site, resulting in the excision of exon 4. This predicts a frameshift in translation with premature protein termination. It remains unclear whether such a truncated variant could exert a dominant negative effect to interfere with the normal functions of wild-type IGF-1 and if the mutation is the cause of the growth retardation. Five other family members with short stature carried wild-type *IGF1*.

Because *IGF1* mutations are extremely rare in the human, all described cases are of considerable interest. Besides a detailed clinical description, thorough biochemical evaluation and genetic analysis, as well as functional experiments are crucial to prove the pathogenicity of the defects and the genotype-phenotype relation.

Molecular *IGF1R* Defects

IGF1R is located on the distal long arm of chromosome 15 (15q26.3) and consists of 21 exons encoding a protein of 1,367 amino acids. The protein is synthesized as a single-chain preproreceptor. After removing the signal peptide, the proreceptor is folded, dimerized by disulfide bonds and glycosylated. Cleavage of the proreceptor results in the mature heterotetrameric ($\alpha_2\beta_2$) transmembrane glycoprotein. The α-subunit is mainly involved in ligand binding, and the β-subunit contains the intracellular tyrosine kinase domain. IGF-1 binds the IGF1R with highest affinity, but IGF-2 and supraphysiological doses of insulin are also able to activate the IGF1R. Ligand binding to the tyrosine kinase receptor results in receptor autophosphorylation on intracellular tyrosine residues and activation of the receptor's intrinsic tyrosine kinase, initiating distinct intracellular signaling pathways [17].

The reported mutations are located throughout the *IGF1R* gene (fig. 2) [6, 18–29]. Besides two compound heterozygous cases [6, 20], only heterozygous carriers have been described. No homozygous mutations have been reported so far. Considering the findings in *IGF1R* null mice, a homozygous *IGF1R* defect in human may not be compatible with life. Based on a clinical suspicion or through screening of a cohort of children born SGA, the reported *IGF1R* defects were identified. In some studies, the pathogenetic relevance of the mutation was supported by the finding that the affected amino acid was an evolutionary highly conserved residue. In most studies, a compromised adult height of carriers of the mutation co-segregated well with the mutation. In addition, the variants were not found in control populations. Ligand

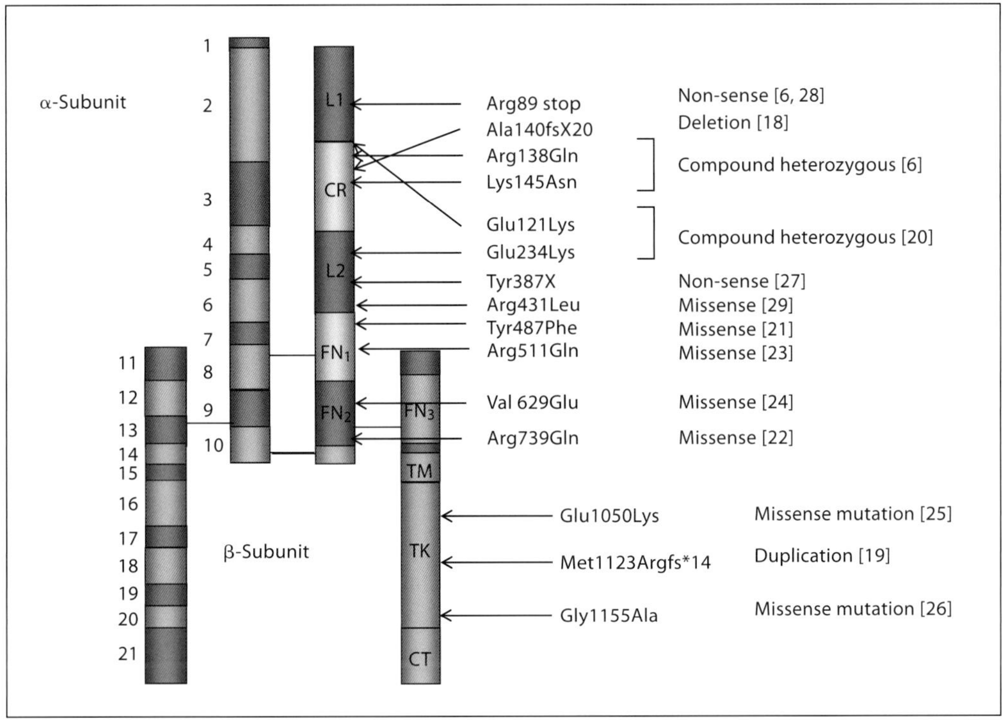

Fig. 2. Heterozygous and compound heterozygous mutations of IGF1R. The 21 exons of *IGF1R* are shown on the left. The domains of the IGF1R protein are on the right. L1/L2 = Leucin rich; CR = cysteine rich; FN = fibronectin; TM = transmembrane; TK = tyrosine kinase; CT = c-terminal. Arg511Gln was published as a pathogenic missense mutation; however, this appears to be a polymorphism as this variant was also found in normal-stature controls.

binding appeared to be reduced in one study [6]. Expression of the IGF1R on the cell surface was reduced in some cases. Functional experiments in fibroblasts of the reported patients or in cellular models showed a decreased autophosphorylation of the β-subunit and subsequently reduced activation of the major signal transduction pathways in all studies. The impairment of cell proliferation was determined by measuring [^{3}H] thymidine incorporation in DNA of fibroblasts or by evaluating the proliferation rate in cells overexpressing the mutant *IGF1R* after a challenge with IGF-1.

From these studies, different mechanisms have been suggested to cause the pathogenicity of the various mutations, including receptor haploinsufficiency, decreased *IGF1R* biosynthesis, interference with ligand binding and transmembrane signaling, and disruption of the intrinsic tyrosine kinase activity [17]. Besides *IGF1R* mutations, also terminal deletions of 15q encompassing *IGF1R* have been reported, which have similar effects of growth and development, but often additional clinical features, such as skeletal and cardiac abnormalities [30].

Similarly to observations in patients with mutations in other genes, the first reported patients with an *IGF1R* defect presented with severe intrauterine growth retardation, postnatal growth failure and microcephaly, while with the publication of more cases, the phenotype appears more variable, presumably depending on the variable pathogenic impact of the mutation (table 2).

The severity of the intrauterine growth retardation appears to be dependent on many factors. In a family with a heterozygous p.Glu1050Lys mutation, we observed a lower birth size in the index patient (birthweight –3.3 SDS, length –4.2 SDS) than in her mother (birthweight –2.1 SDS and length –0.3 SDS) from whom she inherited the mutation [25]. The *IGF1R* of the maternal grandmother was normal, implicating that the mutation was either de novo or of paternal origin. The same pattern was seen in the family with the p.Arg89* mutation described by Abuzzahab et al. [6]. The index case with a mutation of maternal origin had a birthweight of –3.5 SDS and length of –5.8 SDS, while his mother who derived the mutation from her father or de novo had a birthweight of –2.4 SDS and length –1.6 SDS. A proven paternally transmitted mutation of the *IGF1R* resulted in birthweights at the lower limit of the normal range (–2.1 and –1.96 SDS) [18]. This suggests that maternal IGF-1 resistance during pregnancy is one of the factors contributing to the intrauterine growth retardation, possibly by decreased placental growth. This is supported by the finding that decreased IGF1R and signal transduction protein expression is found in placentas from intrauterine growth retardation pregnancies [31].

The most severe postnatal growth retardation (height –7.3 SDS) and microcephaly (–3.8 SDS) was reported in a patient with a compound heterozygous mutation of the *IGF1R* [20]. Interestingly, the parents were both heterozygous for one of the two mutations, but they were phenotypically normal with heights within the normal range (–1.2 and –1.5 SDS) and normal levels of IGF-1, suggesting that haploinsufficiency does not always result in clinically significant IGF-1 resistance.

Biochemically, *IGF1R* defects usually result in serum IGF-1 concentrations above the average for age. However, insufficient feeding can lead to low serum IGF-1. We described a patient with extremely poor appetite and severe failure to thrive [25]. Serum IGF-1 was –0.1 SDS; however, after adequate feeding via a percutaneous gastrostoma IGF-1 increased to +2.9 SDS. Recently, IGF-1 levels of –4.7 SDS were described in a child with a body mass index of –2.6 SDS and a heterozygous p.Tyr487Phe mutation of the IGF1R [21]. IGF-1 level increased to +1.6 SDS during GH treatment and adequate feeding. A low serum IGF-1 was also found in a child with a heterozygous IGF1R deletion in combination with GH deficiency [30].

Data on GH treatment in children with a molecular *IGF1R* defect are limited. So far, 9 patients have been treated with GH [6, 18, 19, 21, 23–25, 29]. Table 3 shows the growth response, which is poor to moderate in most cases. At least one patient had an increase in head circumference during GH treatment [28]. Children treated with GH for the indication born SGA without catch-up growth with a modest growth response

Table 3. Growth response to GH treatment of patients with a heterozygous *IGF1R* mutation

Mutation (protein level)	Reference	Duration of GH treatment	Height
Arg138Gln/Lys145Asn	[6]	10 years (discontinuous)	at 14 years –4.8 SDS
Ala140fs*20 (2 cases)	[18]	11 months 1 year	Δ start-last measured 1.2 SDS Δ start-last measured 0.6 SDS
Arg431Leu	[29]	2 years	Δ start-last measured 0.6 SDS
Tyr487Phe	[21]	4 years	Δ start-last measured 0.8 SDS
Arg511Gln	[23]	6 months	Δ start-last measured 0 SDS
Val629Glu	[24]	11 months	Δ start-last measured 0.1 SDS
Glu1050Lys	[25]	6 8/12 years	Δ start-last measured 0.9 SDS
Met1123Argfs*14	[19]	9 months	no significant catch-up

and unexpected high levels of IGF-1 are good candidates for mutation analysis of *IGF1R*.

In conclusion, molecular defects of the *IGF1* and *IGF1R* gene are rare. The first reports showed severe intrauterine growth and postnatal growth retardation and microcephaly; later reports show a more variable phenotype. Intrauterine growth retardation and microcephaly are not found in patients with GH deficiency or GH resistance, and this can help to find the molecular defect in the GH-IGF-1 axis. Identifying new patients with molecular defects in the GH-IGF-1 axis will help to understand the pathophysiologic mechanisms of impaired IGF-1 action.

References

1 Yakar S, Adamo ML: Insulin-like growth factor 1 physiology: lessons from mouse models. Endocrinol Metab Clin North Am 2012;41:231–247.

2 Lupu F, Terwilliger JD, Lee K, Segre GV, Efstratiadis A: Roles of growth hormone and insulin-like growth factor 1 in mouse postnatal growth. Dev Biol 2001;229:141–162.

3 Woods KA, Camacho-Hübner C, Savage MO, Clark AJ: Intrauterine growth retardation and postnatal growth failure associated with deletion of the insulin-like growth factor I gene. N Engl J Med 1996;335:1363–1367.

4 Liu JP, Baker J, Perkins AS, Robertson EJ, Efstratiadis A: Mice carrying null mutations of the genes encoding insulin-like growth factor I (Igf-1) and type 1 IGF receptor (Igf1r). Cell 1993;75:59–72.

5 Holzenberger M, Leneuve P, Hamard G, Ducos B, Périn L, Binoux M, Le Bouc Y: A targeted partial invalidation of the insulin-like growth factor I receptor gene in mice causes a postnatal growth deficit. Endocrinology 2000;141:2557–2566.

6 Abuzzahab MJ, Schneider A, Goddard A, Grigorescu F, Lautier C, Keller E, Kiess W, Klammt J, Kratzsch J, Osgood D, Pfäffle R, Raile K, Seidel B, Smith RJ, Chernausek SD, Intrauterine Growth Retardation (IUGR) Study Group: IGF-I receptor mutations resulting in intrauterine and postnatal growth retardation. N Engl J Med 2003;349:2211–2222.

7 Woods KA, Camacho-Hübner C, Bergman RN, Barter D, Clark AJ, Savage MO: Effects of insulin-like growth factor I (IGF-I) therapy on body composition and insulin resistance in IGF-I gene deletion. J Clin Endocrinol Metab 2000;85:1407–1411.
8 Bonapace G, Concolino D, Formicola S, Strisciuglio P: A novel mutation in a patient with insulin-like growth factor 1 (IGF1) deficiency. J Med Genet 2003;40:913–917.
9 Concolino D, Muzzi G, Sestito S, Vega G, Bonapace G, Strisciuglio P: Long-term treatment with recombinant insulin-like growth factor 1 (IGF-1) in a child with IGF-1 gene mutation. Eur J Pediatr 2010;169:245–247.
10 Coutinho DC, Coletta RRD, Costa EMF, Pachi PR, Boguszewski MCS, Damiani D, Mendonca BB, Arnhold IJP, Jorge AAL: Polymorphisms identified in the upstream core polyadenylation signal of IGF1 gene exon 6 do not cause pre- and postnatal growth impairment. J Clin Endocrinol Metab 2007;92: 4889–4892.
11 Walenkamp MJE, Karperien M, Pereira AM, et al: Homozygous and heterozygous expression of a novel insulin-like growth factor-I mutation. J Clin Endocrinol Metab 2005;90:2855–2864.
12 Denley A, Wang CC, McNeil KA, Walenkamp MJE, van Duyvenvoorde H, Wit JM, Wallace JC, Norton RS, Karperien M, Forbes BE: Structural and functional characteristics of the Val44Met insulin-like growth factor I missense mutation: correlation with effects on growth and development. Mol Endocrinol 2005;19:711–721.
13 Netchine I, Azzi S, Le Bouc Y, Savage MO: IGF1 molecular anomalies demonstrate its critical role in fetal, postnatal growth and brain development. Best Pract Res Clin Endocrinol Metab 2011;25:181–190.
14 van Duyvenvoorde HA, van Setten PA, Walenkamp MJE, et al: Short stature associated with a novel heterozygous mutation in the insulin-like growth factor 1 gene. J Clin Endocrinol Metab 2010;95: E363–E367.
15 Chellakooty M, Vangsgaard K, Larsen T, Scheike T, Falck-Larsen J, Legarth J, Andersson AM, Main KM, Skakkebaek NE, Juul A: A longitudinal study of intrauterine growth and the placental growth hormone (GH)-insulin-like growth factor I axis in maternal circulation: association between placental GH and fetal growth. J Clin Endocrinol Metab 2004;89:384–391.
16 Fuqua JS, Derr M, Rosenfeld RG, Hwa V: Identification of a novel heterozygous igf1 splicing mutation in a large kindred with familial short stature. Horm Res Paediatr 2012;78:59–66.
17 Klammt J, Kiess W, Pfaffle R: IGF1R mutations as cause of SGA. Best Pract Res Clin Endocrinol Metab 2011;25:191–206.
18 Choi JH, Kang M, Kim GH, Hong M, Jin HY, Lee BH, Park JY, Lee SM, Seo EJ, Yoo HW: Clinical and functional characteristics of a novel heterozygous mutation of the IGF1R gene and IGF1R haploinsufficiency due to terminal 15q26.2->qter deletion in patients with intrauterine growth retardation and postnatal catch-up growth failure. J Clin Endocrinol Metab 2011;96:E130–E134.
19 Fang P, Schwartz ID, Johnson BD, Derr MA, Roberts CT, Hwa V, Rosenfeld RG: Familial short stature caused by haploinsufficiency of the insulin-like growth factor I Receptor due to nonsense-mediated messenger ribonucleic acid decay. J Clin Endocrinol Metab 2009;94:1740–1747.
20 Fang P, Hi Cho Y, Derr MA, Rosenfeld RG, Hwa V, Cowell CT: Severe short stature caused by novel compound heterozygous mutations of the insulin-like growth factor 1 receptor (IGF1R). J Clin Endocrinol Metab 2012;97:E243–E247.
21 Labarta JI, Barrio E, Audí L, Fernández-Cancio M, Andaluz P, de Arriba A, Puga B, Calvo MT, Mayayo E, Carrascosa A, Ferrández-Longás A: Familial short stature and intrauterine growth retardation associated with a novel mutation in the IGF-I receptor (IGF1R) gene. Clin Endocrinol (Oxf) 2012, Epub ahead of print.
22 Kawashima Y: Mutation at cleavage site of insulin-like growth factor receptor in a short-stature child born with intrauterine growth retardation. J Clin Endocrinol Metab 2005;90:4679–4687.
23 Inagaki K, Tiulpakov A, Rubtsov P, Sverdlova P, Peterkova V, Yakar S, Terekhov S, LeRoith D: A familial insulin-like growth factor-I receptor mutant leads to short stature: clinical and biochemical characterization. J Clin Endocrinol Metab 2007; 92:1542–1548.
24 Wallborn T, Wuller S, Klammt J, Kruis T, Kratzsch J, Schmidt G, Schlicke M, Muller E, Schmitz van de Leur H, Kiess W, Pfaffle R: A heterozygous mutation of the insulin-like growth factor-I receptor causes retention of the nascent protein in the endoplasmic reticulum and results in intrauterine and postnatal growth retardation. J Clin Endocrinol Metab 2010;95:2316–2324.
25 Walenkamp MJE, van der Kamp HJ, Pereira AM, Kant SG, van Duyvenvoorde HA, Kruithof MF, Breuning MH, Romijn JA, Karperien M, Wit JM: A variable degree of intrauterine and postnatal growth retardation in a family with a missense mutation in the insulin-like growth factor I receptor. J Clin Endocrinol Metab 2006;91:3062–3070.

26 Kruis T, Klammt J, Galli-Tsinopoulou A, Wallborn T, Schlicke M, Muller E, Kratzsch J, Korner A, Odeh R, Kiess W, Pfaffle R: Heterozygous mutation within a kinase-conserved motif of the insulin-like growth factor I receptor causes intrauterine and postnatal growth retardation. J Clin Endocrinol Metab 2010;95:1137–1142.
27 Mohn A, Marcovecchio ML, de Giorgis T, Pfaeffle R, Chiarelli F, Kiess W: An insulin-like growth factor-I receptor defect associated with short stature and impaired carbohydrate homeostasis in an Italian pedigree. Horm Res Paediatr 2011;76:136–143.
28 Raile K, Klammt J, Schneider A, Keller A, Laue S, Smith R, Pfaffle R, Kratzsch J, Keller E, Kiess W: Clinical and functional characteristics of the human Arg59Ter insulin-like growth factor I receptor (IGF1R) mutation: implications for a gene dosage effect of the human IGF1R. J Clin Endocrinol Metab 2006;91:2264–2271.
29 Kawashima Y, Higaki K, Fukushima T, Hakuno F, Nagaishi J-I, Hanaki K, Nanba E, Takahashi S-I, Kanzaki S: Novel missense mutation in the IGF-I receptor L2 domain results in intrauterine and postnatal growth retardation. Clin Endocrinol (Oxf) 2012;77:246–254.
30 Ester WA, van Duyvenvoorde HA, de Wit CC, Broekman AJ, Ruivenkamp CAL, Govaerts LCP, Wit JM, Hokken-Koelega ACS, Losekoot M: Two short children born small for gestational age with insulin-like growth factor 1 receptor haploinsufficiency illustrate the heterogeneity of its phenotype. J Clin Endocrinol Metab 2009;94:4717–4727.
31 Laviola L, Perrini S, Belsanti G, Natalicchio A, Montrone C, Leonardini A, Vimercati A, Scioscia M, Selvaggi L, Giorgino R, Greco P, Giorgino F: Intrauterine growth restriction in humans is associated with abnormalities in placental insulin-like growth factor signaling. Endocrinology 2005;146: 1498–1505.
32 Netchine I, Azzi S, Houang M, Seurin D, Perin L, Ricort J-M, Daubas C, Legay C, Mester J, Herich R, Godeau F, Le Bouc Y: Partial primary deficiency of insulin-like growth factor (IGF)-I activity associated with IGF1 mutation demonstrates its critical role in growth and brain development. J Clin Endocrinol Metab 2009;94:3913–3921.

M.J.E. Walenkamp, MD, PhD
Department of Pediatrics, 9D11, VU University Medical Center
De Boelelaan 1117
NL–1081 HV Amsterdam (The Netherlands)
E-Mail m.walenkamp@vumc.nl

Maghnie M, Loche S, Cappa M, Ghizzoni L, Lorini R (eds): Hormone Resistance and Hypersensitivity. From Genetics to Clinical Management. Endocr Dev. Basel, Karger, 2013, vol 24, pp 138–149 (DOI: 10.1159/000342578)

Phenotypes, Investigation and Treatment of Primary IGF-1 Deficiency

Martin O. Savage

Department of Endocrinology, William Harvey Research Institute, Barts and the London School of Medicine and Dentistry, London, UK

Abstract

GH insensitivity, also known as primary IGF-1 deficiency (PIGFD), presents as growth failure, and in its severe form is associated with dysmorphic and metabolic abnormalities. PIGFD is caused by genetic defects in the GH-IGF-1 axis. The field of PIGFD due to mutations affecting GH action has evolved since the original description of the extreme phenotype related to homozygous GH receptor mutations over 40 years ago. A continuum of genetic, phenotypic, and biochemical abnormalities can be defined associated with clinically relevant defects in linear growth. A systematic protocol of investigation assessing Gh secretion and the IGF system will lead to a diagnosis of PIGFD. PIGFD can be effectively treated with rhIGF-1, the optimal recommended maintenance dose being 120 μg/kg twice daily by SC injection. Most therapeutic experience is in severely affected patients with the Laron syndrome phenotype, who show growth acceleration and may reach normal adult height. Further controlled studies are needed in more mildly affected subjects.

GH insensitivity (GHI; OMIM No. 262500 and 245590) was first reported by Laron [1] in 1966, with the description of 3 children with extreme growth failure from a consanguineous Jewish family of Yemenite origin who had the phenotype of hypopituitarism with high serum GH concentrations. Although an abnormal GH molecule was initially suspected, this disorder, for many years referred to as Laron syndrome, was shown to be caused by a defect in the GH receptor (GHR) [2]. This striking but very rare phenotype, which was also untreatable at that time, became synonymous with the diagnosis of primary IGF-1 deficiency (PIGFD). In the late 1980s, two pivotal developments brought important changes to the field. The first was the synthesis and availability of recombinant human IGF-1 for therapy [3] and the second was the advent of molecular techniques, which led to the cloning and characterization of the human *GHR* [4].

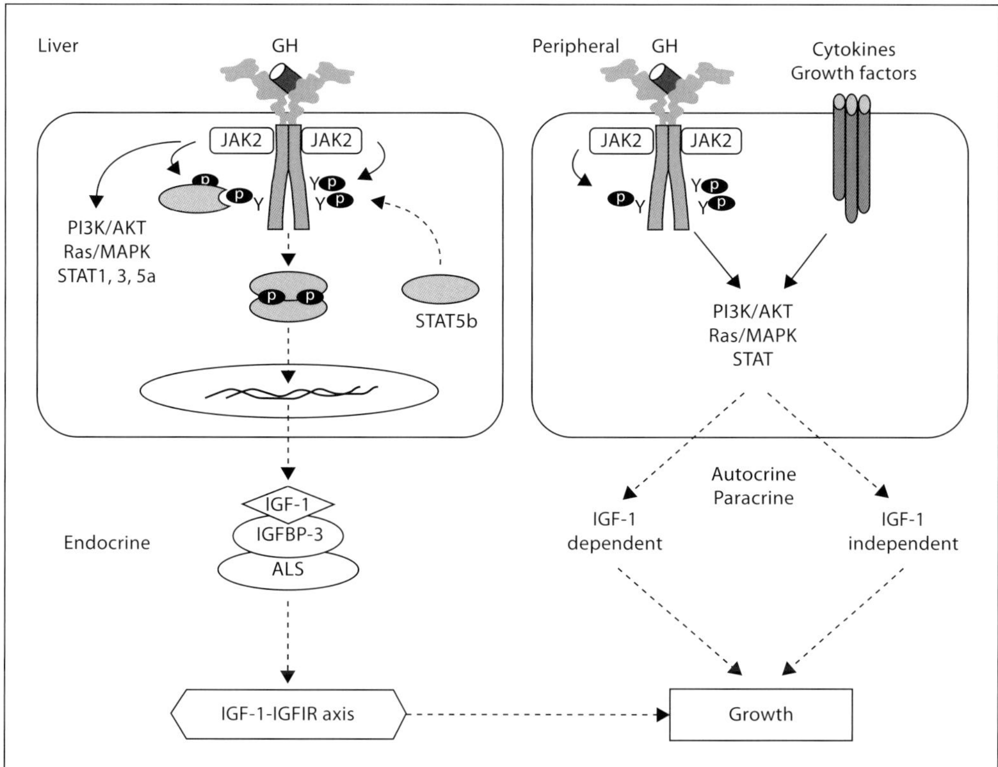

Fig. 1. The GH-IGF-1 axis in human growth. Solid arrows indicate activation processes, dashed arrows, translocation processes. P = Phosphorylated residue; Y = tyrosine; AKT = v-akt murine thymoma viral oncogene homolog, also known as PKB, protein kinase B; ALS = acid labile subunit; MAPK = mitogen-activated protein kinase; PI3K = phosphatidylinositol 3-kinase.

PIGFD is not a single entity, but a broad diagnostic category comprising a range of molecular defects in the GH-IGF axis. These defects, which may involve genes coding for proteins that regulate GH binding or signal transduction and IGF-1 synthesis, transport or action, are associated with an equally varied range of phenotypes and biochemical abnormalities. This chapter will describe the range of phenotypes and the investigation of possible PIGFD and summarise its treatment with rhIGF-1.

Physiology of GH and the IGF-1 System in Relation to Linear Growth

The actions of GH are mediated by a combination of components of the IGF system, including IGF-1, IGF-binding proteins (IGFBPs), the IGF-1 receptor (IGFIR), and IGF-independent effects through direct GH action. A diagram of the GH-IGF axis is shown in figure 1. Following the original 'somatomedin hypothesis' [5], in 1985 Green et al. [6] proposed the 'dual effector hypothesis' suggesting that GH regulates the expression of locally produced IGF-1, which then acts in an autocrine/paracrine manner. Expression of the *IGF1* gene was found in multiple tissues throughout embryonic and postnatal development. In addition, injection of GH into hypophysectomised rats increased *IGF1* mRNA in numerous non-hepatic tissues. Direct injection of GH into the cartilage growth plate of hypophysectomised rats also resulted in significantly increased longitudinal bone growth [7]. Hence, GH has local effects, independent of those mediated by circulating IGF-1. Nilsson et al. [8] demonstrated that GH stimulated differentiation of preadipocytes and chondrocytes in the growth plate, while IGF-1 stimulated their clonal expansion.

Le Roith et al. [9] took account of gene deletion experiments in mice to question the role of liver-derived IGF-1 in controlling postnatal growth and development. Liver-specific *Igf1* knockout mice grow normally despite reduction in circulating IGF-1, indicating that locally produced IGF-1 was an important growth mediator [9]. Some 75% of serum IGF-1 is liver derived, while the remainder originates from non-hepatic tissues. In addition, serum levels of the acid-labile subunit (ALS) and IGFBP-3 are important in maintaining circulating IGF-1 [10]. The importance of ALS was clearly shown in the *Igfals* knockout mouse model and by Domené et al. [11] who reported the first homozygous mutation in human *IGFALS* causing severe IGF-1 deficiency.

Mechanisms of GH and IGF-1 Actions

Pituitary-derived GH exerts its growth effects primarily by regulating the expression of IGF-1 (fig. 1). GH regulates IGF-1 production through the STAT (signal transducer and activator of transcription)-5b signalling system. The binding of GH to the cell surface homodimeric GHR recruits and induces signal transduction through the cytosolic Janus kinase 2 (JAK2). Initiation of signal transduction through the STAT5b pathway requires STAT5b to associate with one of several JAK2 phosphorylated tyrosines located on the intracellular domain of GHR. STAT5b, recruited to GH-activated GHR, is subsequently phosphorylated by JAK2, whereupon the tyrosyl-phosphorlated-STAT5b forms a homodimer and translocates to the nucleus. The dimeric phosphorylated STAT5b binds to chromosomal GH responsive elements and drives transcriptional regulations of STAT5b-dependent genes [12].

IGF-1 produced in the liver circulates in a ternary complex with liver-derived IGFBP-3 and ALS, and is delivered to IGF-1-responsive cells and tissues. The mitogenic and metabolic effects of IGF-1 are mediated through the type I IGFIR, a cell-surface tyrosine kinase receptor encoded by *IGF1R*. The binding of IGF-1 to IGFIR leads to receptor autophosphorylation, resulting in recruitment of cytoplasmic

Table 1. Classification of GHI and PIGFD disorders with short stature

Defects of the GH-IGF-1 axis
1. GHR defects
a. Extracellular mutations
b. Transmembrane mutations
c. Intracellular mutations
2. GH signal transduction defects (STAT5b)
3. Mutations of SHP-2 (encoded by *PTPN11*), K-RAS, H-RAS
4. *IGF1* gene mutations or deletions
a. Defects causing IGF-1 deficiency
b. Bio-inactive IGF-1
5. ALS defects
6. *IGFIR* gene mutations
7. GH-neutralizing antibodies in patients with *GH* gene deletion

PTPN11 = Protein tyrosine phosphatase, nonreceptor type 11; SHP-2 = Src homology region 2-domain phosphatase-2.

components of downstream signalling pathways, including the PI3K/Akt and MAPK/Erk pathways, ultimately leading to cell proliferation and other metabolic effects [12].

Phenotypes of Primary IGF-1 Deficiency Caused by Human GH-IGF Axis Mutations

Normal GH secretion and the functional integrity of the IGF system are essential for normal linear growth. Defects that have been identified to cause impaired growth are shown in table 1. A summary of phenotypic and biochemical features in the range of GH-IGF-1 axis defects is given in table 2. Human prenatal growth is regulated principally by nutritional supplies, which influence fetal IGF-1 [13]. The importance of normal IGF-1 production in humans was confirmed by the prenatal growth failure reported in patients with *IGF1* mutations [14, 15]. IGF-1 action is also essential as demonstrated by humans with mutations of *IGF1R* [12]. Postnatal growth may be disrupted by mutations that disturb the functional integrity of the cascade of GH-GHR interaction, GH signal transduction, and IGF-1 production, transport and action [12].

The Continuum of Phenotypic Features

The concept of genotype:phenotype relationships in endocrinology can be applied to defects of the GH-IGF axis causing PIGFD. Since populations of children with PIGFD were first reported, a range of phenotypes has been described. This was

Table 2. Summary of phenotypic and biochemical features in the range of GH-IGF-1 axis defects.

Phenotype	Gene defect							
	GHR	*STAT5b*	*PTPN11*	*IGF-1*	*IGFALS*	*IGFIR*	Bio-inactive GH	*GH1* with anti-GH antibodies
Severe growth failure	+/–	+	–	+	–	–	–	+
Mild growth failure	–/+	–	+	–	+	+	+	–
Mid-face hypoplasia	+/–	+/–	–	–	–	–	–	+
Other facial dysmorphism	–	–	+	+	–	+	–	–
Deafness	–	–	–	+	–	–	–	–
Microcephaly	–	–	–	+	–	+	–	–
Intellectual delay	–	–	–/+	+	–	+/–	–	–
Puberty delay	+/–	+/–	+/–	–	+	–	–	–
Immune deficiency	–	+	–	–	–	–	–	–
Hypoglycaemia	+	–/+	–	–	–	–	–	–
Hyperinsulinaemia	–	–	-	+	+	–	–	–
IGF-1 deficiency	+	+	–/+	+/–	+	–	+	+
IGFBP-3 deficiency	+	+	–/+	–	+	–	+	+
ALS deficiency	+	+	–/+	–	+	–	+	+
GH excess	+	+	–	+/–	+	–	–	–
GHBP deficiency	+/–	–	–	–	–	–	–	–
Homozygous or compound heterozygous mutations	+	+	–	+	+	–	–/+	+
Heterozygous mutations	–	–	+	–	–	+	+/–	_

+ = Positive; – = negative; +/– = predominantly positive; –/+ = predominantly negative; GHBP = growth hormone-binding protein.

noticeable in the series of 82 patients, mainly of European origin, who were identified in the early 1990s for rhIGF-1 therapy [16]. There was a gradation of severity of short stature, with height standard deviation score (SDS) ranging from –2.2 to –10.4 and a strong positive correlation ($r^2 = 0.45$, $p \leq 0.001$) between height SDS and IGFBP-3 SDS. A further variable in the same population related to phenotype was the serum GHBP level which when very low or absent was associated with more severe short stature (height SDS –6.45) whilst normal GHBP values were associated with milder short stature (height SDS –4.89) [16]. A study of craniofacial phenotype in the same group of subjects identified that those with normal facial appearance had milder short stature and could present as idiopathic short stature [12]. However in this series of GH-resistant patients, there was no clear relationship between *GHR* mutation and phenotype [16]. In patients from Ecuador with the homozygous E180 splice *GHR* mutation, heterogeneity of statural phenotype was also seen with height SDS values ranging from –5.3 to –11.5 and height SDS correlated positively ($p < 0.01$) with both IGF-1 SDS and IGFBP-3 SDS values [12].

GHR Mutations

Thirty-eight patients with PIGFD were studied in the Centre for Endocrinology at Barts and the London School of Medicine and Dentistry, London, and identified to have homozygous, compound heterozygous or heterozygous dominant negative *GHR* mutations [12]. In order to perform an assessment of height SDS and type of *GHR* mutation, these 38 subjects were analysed together with 32 subjects, also fulfilling the same PIGFD criteria, who were added from the literature. Relationships between *GHR* mutation type and height SDS are shown in figure 2. For the first time, dominant negative *GHR* mutations [17] and *GHR* intronic pseudoexon mutations [18] were associated with significantly less severe growth phenotypes ($p < 0.05$) than *GHR* missense and non-sense mutations.

STAT5B and IGFALS Mutations

Patients with homozygous *STAT5B* mutations have a range of phenotypic characteristics [12]. Height SDS values ranged from –5.6 to –9.9. The majority of these patients had serious immunological abnormalities, which almost certainly contributed to their growth failure. In a recent review of 17 cases with homozygous *IGFALS* mutations, height SDS values in prepubertal subjects ($n = 15$) ranged from –1.1 to –3.9 (mean –2.6), in adolescent subjects ($n = 10$) from –1.0 to –4.4 (mean –2.8) and in adult subjects ($n = 8$) from –0.5 to –4.4 (mean –2.2) [19].

IGF1 Mutations

The key feature of *IGF1* defects is their association with impaired fetal growth. Key additional phenotypic features of *IGF1* defects are microcephaly, deafness, and some degree of intellectual retardation [14, 15]. However, as more cases are diagnosed, the phenotype is likely to evolve.

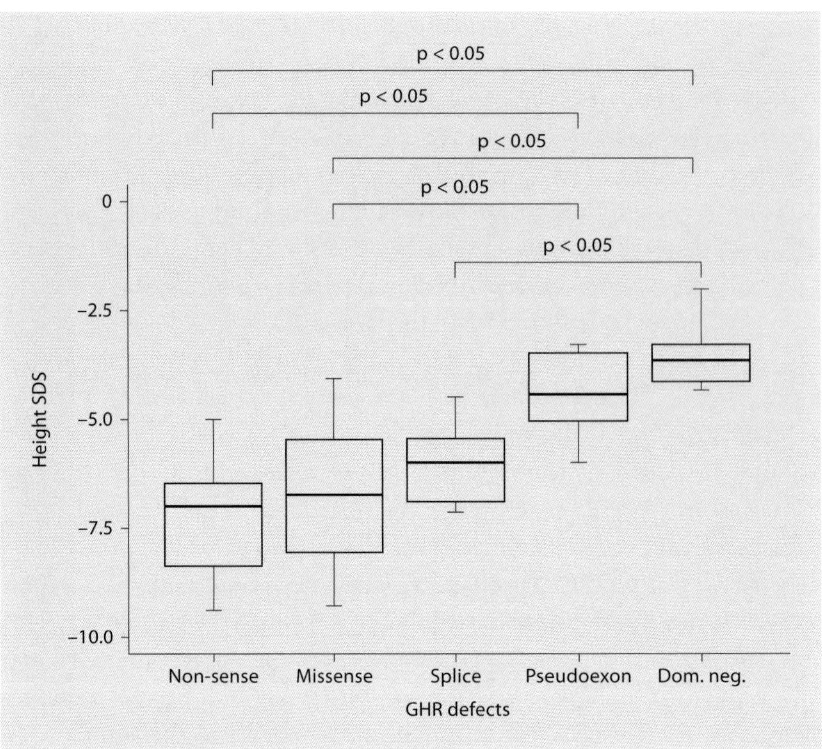

Fig. 2. Height SDS values in 70 children with PIGFD and *GHR* mutations divided according to the type of mutation [12]. Each boxplot depicts the median, 25th and 75th percentiles. Whiskers depict minimum and maximum observed values. Statistical analyses were performed using R version 2.6.2 (R Development Core Team, 2008, R Foundation for Statistical Computing, Vienna, Austria). Numerical variables were expressed as median (range). Comparison between continuous variables was performed using the Student's t test. A two-sided p value <0.05 was considered indicative of statistical significance. Bonferroni adjustment was performed to reduce the likelihood of type I error.

The Continuum of Biochemical Changes

The cardinal features of PIGFD states are deficiency of IGF-1 and normal or increased GH secretion. In *GHR* mutations, IGF-1, IGFBP-3, and ALS levels are usually severely decreased, although the degree is variable [12]. Most homozygous *GHR* mutations cause extreme deficiency of all GH-dependent peptides with increase in basal and stimulated GH secretion [16]. However, a range of IGF-1 and IGFBP-3 deficiencies was present particularly in some of the less homogeneous populations where a range of IGFBP-3 values was noticeable. A range of IGF-1 deficiency was also present in patients from Ecuador [12]. Patients with dominant negative, splice site and the pseudoexon 6Ψ *GHR* mutations have a less severe IGF-1 deficiency compared to PIGFD subjects with non-sense and *GHR* missense mutations [12].

GHR Mutations

In the recent study of PIGFD cases with identified *GHR* mutations performed at St Bartholomew's Hospital, serum IGF-1 levels were available in 41 subjects [12]. A range of IGF-1 deficiency was demonstrated in association with different *GHR* mutations. IGF-1 SDS values were lower ($p < 0.05$) in subjects with missense and non-sense *GHR* mutations than in those with the pseudoexon mutations, as previously described [12]. Patients with *GHR* splice site mutations and dominant negative defects had higher ($p < 0.05$) IGF-1 levels than subjects with missense mutations. These findings show that a continuum of IGF-1 levels exists across the spectrum of *GHR* mutations reflecting the degree of receptor dysfunction.

STAT5B and IGFALS Mutations

STAT5B mutations are associated with severe PIGFD, reflected in marked deficiencies of all GH-dependent peptides and increase in GH secretion [20]. In subjects with homozygous *IGFALS* mutations, serum ALS levels are almost universally undetectable, and failure to form the circulating ternary complex results in rapid clearance and extreme deficiency of IGF-1 and ALS [12, 19]. In a recent review by Domené et al. [19], serum IGF-1 SDS values ranged from –3.2 to –11.2 and IGFBP-3 SDS values from –3.6 to –18.5. GH secretion was increased in the majority of subjects, which may contribute to some degree of insulin resistance [12].

IGF1 Mutations

In the four cases with homozygous *IGF1* defects and the patients with a heterozygous mutation causing a definite growth phenotype, serum IGF-1 levels varied according to the nature of the mutation. IGFBP-3 and ALS levels were notably normal, and GH secretion was usually normal or increased [15].

Investigation of Primary IGF-1 Deficiency

The evaluation of a child with possible PIGFD should comply with the classical paradigm of clinical assessment followed by general (i.e. non-endocrine) investigations, hormonal assessment, and possible genetic analyses. As advances in molecular endocrinology progress, the importance of detailed phenotypic evaluation and documentation becomes increasingly appreciated. Clinical assessment should include enquiries about family history of growth disturbance, consanguinity, birthweight and length, and recurrent infections [12]. Examination should specifically assess the presence of possible facial dysmorphic features and microcephaly in addition to anthropometric evaluation.

Investigations of the GH-IGF-1 axis consist of determination of GH secretion and exploration of the IGF system. A GH provocation test is recommended unless the child has normal auxology or a basal IGF-1 level above the mean for age. In a child with clinical criteria of GHD, a peak GH level of <10 ng/ml has traditionally been used to support this diagnosis. Basal IGF-1 levels should also be determined, although these may be influenced by factors such as age, nutrition, chronic illness, and puberty. In the initial assessment, IGFBP-3 adds little, except in children under 3 years of age, where low IGFBP-3 is helpful in the diagnosis of GHD. Reliable assay performance and appropriate normative data [21] are essential for the use of IGF-1 and IGFBP-3 in clinical practice, and adjustment for sex, age, puberty, and nutritional status is recommended.

A diagnosis of PIGFD follows from the demonstration of abnormal auxology, normal GH secretion, and IGF-1 deficiency [12]. However, the pathogenesis will not have been elucidated from these investigations. The nature of the defect can often be defined by additional measurement of IGFBP-3, ALS, and GHBP [12].

The principle behind the design of the IGF-1 generation test (IGFGT) was that repeated injections of hGH induce measurable increases in IGF-1, IGFBP-3, and ALS secretion. Interest in the IGFGT was renewed when subjects were selected for rhIGF-1 therapy. A recent review has critically appraised the value of the IGFGT in paediatric endocrine practice [22]. Criteria for diagnosis of PIGFD were defined as: failure to increase IGF-1 and IGFBP-3 by >15 and 400 ng/ml, respectively [16]. However, these criteria now appear to be too strict for more mildly affected subjects. Attempts to refine the IGFGT for the diagnosis of milder GHI have demonstrated that patients with idiopathic short stature produced a subnormal response and subjects with IGF-1 deficiency and normal GH secretion also had subnormal ability to generate IGF-1 [12]. Additional sensitivity for the diagnosis of GH resistance was not seen with a low-dose GH protocol and a lack of reproducibility of IGF-1 and IGFBP-3 responses in the test has also been reported [22]. The principal value of the IGFGT is the confirmation of extreme or severe GHI [22].

Genetic Investigations

Single gene mutations in the GH-IGF-1 axis make a major contribution to the pathogenesis of PIGFD. Following clinical and biochemical assessment and where a genetic cause of short stature is expected from the family history, DNA analysis for key candidate genes can confirm a genetic diagnosis. A hierarchy and priority of molecular tests can be defined following careful clinical and biochemical assessment. Testing for molecular defects in the GH-IGF-1 axis is not commercially available at the present time. However, a number of academic laboratories perform DNA sequencing studies of the relevant candidate genes. In vitro functional studies may also be necessary to quantitate the degree of protein dysfunction, particularly in cases with a milder phenotype. There are many components of the GH and IGF signalling cascades that remain poorly understood and are legitimate candidates for harbouring significant mutations and/or deletions. Thus, the absence of identifiable mutations in the candidate genes described above cannot rule out the possibility of a molecular abnormality of the GH-IGF axis.

Ideally, family members should also be tested. It is now clear that members of a family with the same mutations may have differing phenotypes. Additionally, for many of the autosomal recessive disorders described above, the issue of heterozygous expression remains of great interest and warrants further study [23].

Treatment of Primary IGF-1 Deficiency

PIGFD may be diagnosed in some patients labelled as idiopathic short stature [24]. Such patients would not be expected to have a favourable response to treatment with GH. Consequently, treatment with rhIGF-1 may have a place in their management [24]. IGF-1 therapy was initiated in the late 1980s, but supplies were irregular, and it is only recently that guaranteed supplies have become available.

Early trials of IGF-1 therapy in severe GH resistance mostly caused by GHR defects demonstrated a growth-promoting effect when IGF-1 was administered in a dose of 80–120 μg/kg/dose twice daily [25, 26]. The largest body of long-term growth data came from the accumulated experience of patients treated for up to 12 years in North America [26]. These data were submitted to the FDA, and in 2005 rhIGF-1 was approved for treatment of severe PIGFD, defined as serum IGF-1 <–3 SD, height <–3 SD and normal GH concentrations. Approval for the same indication (IGF-1 <2.5th centile) was obtained by the European Medicines Evaluation Agency in 2007.

The spectrum of GH resistance is wider than the small group of patients with homozygous single gene defects. Major diagnostic challenges exist related to the nature and scope of the molecular defects causing short stature, with poor long-term height prognosis, and fulfilling FDA and EMEA labels. The optimal management of this broad range of patients also needs to be established. Controlled therapeutic trials with IGF-1 in patients with IGF-1 deficiency have shown a range of growth responses for which further analysis will indicate which patients would be expected to benefit most [24].

Conclusions

From the fundamental importance of the GH-IGF axis in human linear growth, it follows that defects at many points in this axis will result in growth impairment leading to childhood and adult short stature. The key defects leading to PIGFD have been described, and the range of genetic, clinical, and biochemical abnormalities, both within each genetic disorder and within the spectrum of PIGFD disorders as a whole has been emphasised. GHI can no longer be considered to be a single clinical entity, as it was envisaged nearly 50 years ago. As new genetic defects leading to an expansion of the field of PIGFD are described, each new mutation will itself contribute to the genetic and phenotypic continuum.

Treatment with rhIGF-1 provides an opportunity for children with PIGFD to grow and ultimately reach a normal height. Experience of treatment of mildly affected patients remains limited and requires further controlled studies. However, rhIGF-1 has true promise as a therapeutic modality, and its potential is likely to be further demonstrated in the coming decade.

References

1 Laron Z: Laron syndrome (primary growth hormone resistance or insensitivity): the personal experience 1958–2003. J Clin Endocrinol Metab 2004; 89:1031–1044.

2 Eshet R, Laron Z, Pertzelan A, Arnon R, Dintzman M: Defect of human growth hormone receptors in the liver of two patients with Laron-type dwarfism. Isr J Med Sci 1984;20:8–11.

3 Laron Z, Klinger B, Erster B, Anin S: Effect of acute administration of insulin-like growth factor I in patients with Laron-type dwarfism. Lancet 1988; 2:1170–1172.

4 Godowski PJ, Leung DW, Meacham LR, Galgani JP, Hellmiss R, Keret R, Rotwein PS, Parks JS, Laron Z, Wood WI: Characterization of the human growth hormone receptor gene and demonstration of a partial gene deletion in two patients with Laron-type dwarfism. Proc Natl Acad Sci U S A 1989;86: 8083–8087.

5 Salmon WD Jr, Daughaday WH: A hormonally controlled serum factor which stimulates sulphate incorporation by cartilage in vitro. J Lab Clin Med 1957;49:825–836.

6 Green H, Morikawa M, Nixon T: A dual effector theory of growth-hormone action. Differentiation 1985;29:195–198.

7 Isaksson OG, Jansson JO, Gause IA: Growth hormone stimulates longitudinal bone growth directly. Science 1982;216:1237–1239.

8 Nilsson A, Isgaard J, Lindahl A, Dahlstrom A, Skottner A, Isaksson OG: Regulation by growth hormone of number of chondrocytes containing IGF-I in rat growth plate. Science 1986;233:571–574.

9 Le Roith D, Bondy C, Yakar S, Liu JL, Butler A: The somatomedin hypothesis: 2001. Endocr Rev 2001; 22:53–74.

10 Ohlsson C, Mohan S, Sjögren K, Tivesten A, Isgaard J, Isaksson O, Jansson JO, Svensson J: The role of liver-derived insulin-like growth factor-I. Endocr Rev 2009;30:494–535.

11 Domené HM, Bengolea SV, Martínez AS, Ropelato MG, Pennisi P, Scaglia P, Heinrich JJ, Jasper HG: Deficiency of the circulating insulin-like growth factor system associated with inactivation of the acid-labile subunit gene. N Engl J Med 2004;350: 570–577.

12 David A, Hwa V, Metherell LA, Netchine I, Camacho-Hübner C, Clark AJL, Rosenfeld RG, Savage MO: Evidence for a continuum of genetic, phenotypic and biochemical abnormalities in children with growth hormone insensitivity. Endocr Rev 2011;32:472–497.

13 Fowden AL: The insulin-like growth factors and feto-placental growth. Placenta 2003;24:803–812.

14 Woods KA, Camacho-Hübner C, Savage MO, Clark AJL: Intrauterine growth retardation and post-natal growth failure associated with deletion of the insulin-like growth factor-I gene. N Engl J Med 1996;335:1363–1367.

15 Netchine I, Azzi S, Le Bouc Y, Savage MO: IGF1 molecular anomalies demonstrate its critical role in fetal, postnatal growth and brain development. Best Pract Res Clin Endocrinol Metab 2011;25:181–190.

16 Woods KA, Dastot F, Preece MA, Clark AJL, Postel-Vinay MC, Chatelain PG, Ranke MB, Rosenfeld RG, Amselem S, Savage MO: Phenotype: genotype relationships in growth hormone insensitivity syndrome. J Clin Endocrinol Metab 1997;82:3529–3535.

17 Ayling RM, Ross R, Towner P, Von Laue S, Finidori J, Moutoussamy S, Buchanan CR, Clayton PE, Norman MR: A dominant-negative mutation of the growth hormone receptor causes familial short stature. Nat Genet 1997;16:3–14.
18 Metherell LA, Akker SA, Munroe PB, Rose SJ, Caulfield M, Savage MO, Chew SL, Clark AJL: Pseudoexon activation as a novel mechanism for disease resulting in atypical growth hormone insensitivity. Am J Hum Genet 2001;69:641–646.
19 Domené HM, Hwa V, Argente J, Wit JM, Camacho-Hübner C, Jasper HG, Pozo J, van Duyvenvoorde HA, Yakar S, Fofanova-Gambetti OV, Rosenfeld RG; International ALS Collaborative Group: Human acid-labile subunit deficiency: clinical, endocrine and metabolic consequences. Horm Res Pediatr 2009;72:129–141.
20 Rosenfeld RG, Belgorosky A, Camacho-Hubner C, Savage MO, Wit JM, Hwa V: Defects in growth hormone receptor signaling. Trends Endocrinol Metab 2007;18:134–141.
21 Juul A, Bang P, Hertel NT, Main K, Dalgaard P, Jørgensen K, Müller J, Hall K, Skakkebaek NE: Serum insulin-like growth factor-I in 1030 healthy children, adolescents and adults: relation to age, sex, stage of puberty, testicular size and body mass index. J Clin Endocrinol Metab 1994;78:744–752.
22 Coutant R, Dörr HG, Gleeson H, Argente J: Limitations of the IGF-I generation test in children with short stature. Eur J Endocrinol 2011;166:351–357.
23 Fofanova-Gambetti OV, Hwa V, Wit JM, Domene HM, Argente J, Bang P, Högler W, Kirsch S, Pihoker C, Chiu HK, Cohen L, Jacobsen C, Jasper HG, Haeusler G, Campos-Barros A, Gallego-Gómez E, Gracia-Bouthelier R, van Duyvenvoorde HA, Pozo J, Rosenfeld RG: Impact of heterozygosity for acid-labile subunit (IGFALS) gene mutations on stature: results from the international acid-labile subunit consortium. J Clin Endocrinol Metab 2010;95:4184–4191.
24 Midyett LK, Rogol AD, Frane J, Bright GM: Recombinant insulin-like growth factor (IGF)-I treatment in short children with low IGF-I levels: first-year results from a randomised clinical trial J Clin Endocrinol Metab 2009;95:611–619.
25 Ranke MB, Savage MO, Chatelain PG, Preece MA, Rosenfeld RG, Wilton P: Long-term treatment of growth hormone insensitivity syndrome with IGF-I. Results of the European Multicentre Study. The Working Group on Growth Hormone Insensitivity Syndromes. Horm Res 1999;51:128–134.
26 Chernausek SD, Backeljauw PF, Frane J, Kuntze J, Underwood LE: Long-term treatment with recombinant insulin-like growth factor (IGF)-I in children with severe IGF-I deficiency due to growth hormone insensitivity. J Clin Endocrinol Metab 2007;92:902–910.

Prof. Martin O. Savage
Department of Endocrinology, William Harvey Research Institute
Barts and the London School of Medicine & Dentistry, John Vane Science Centre
Charterhouse Square, London EC1M 6BQ (UK)
E-Mail m.o.savage@qmul.ac.uk

Maghnie M, Loche S, Cappa M, Ghizzoni L, Lorini R (eds): Hormone Resistance and Hypersensitivity. From Genetics to Clinical Management. Endocr Dev. Basel, Karger, 2013, vol 24, pp 150–155 (DOI: 10.1159/000342511)

Human Congenital Perilipin Deficiency and Insulin Resistance

Kristina Kozusko · Satish Patel · David B. Savage

Metabolic Research Laboratories, Institute of Metabolic Science, University of Cambridge, Addenbrooke's Hospital, Cambridge, UK

Abstract

Lipid droplets (LDs) can form in all eukaryotic cells, but white adipocytes are uniquely adapted to store energy as neutral lipid within a large unilocular LD. Non-esterified fatty acids can then be released from the LD store by lipases for use in oxidative tissues. Perilipin was the first mammalian LD protein to be identified in adipocytes where it plays a key role in co-ordinating access of lipases to the core triacylglycerol. We recently identified the first human loss-of-function mutations in PLIN1 in patients with a novel form of familial partial lipodystrophy, severe insulin resistance, diabetes, dyslipidaemia and fatty liver. Adipose tissue samples from affected patients revealed remarkably similar features to those previously observed in samples from obese insulin resistant patients, namely macrophage infiltration and fibrosis. Cellular mechanistic studies suggest that the mutations lead to increased basal lipolysis, which is likely to be a major factor in the subsequent inflammatory response. Perilipin is almost exclusively expressed in white adipocytes, so the serious metabolic sequelae observed in these patients suggest that primary defects in adipose tissue can lead to all the typical features seen in patients with the metabolic syndrome. They also suggest that lipolytic inhibitors may be therapeutically useful in these patients.

Insulin resistance (IR), usually defined as a reduction in the ability of a given concentration of insulin to lower blood glucose levels, underpins the tight associations between obesity and type 2 diabetes (T2DM), dyslipidaemia, atherosclerosis, polycystic ovarian syndrome and non-alcoholic fatty liver disease (NAFLD). Interestingly, lipodystrophy, which is characterised by a paucity of adipose tissue rather than an excess, is associated with severe IR and almost identical metabolic problems to those usually associated with too much fat, i.e. obesity. This paradox highlights the pivotal contribution of adipose tissue in maintaining healthy metabolic homeostasis.

Lipodystrophies

Lipodystrophies are a heterogeneous group of disorders characterised by a selective loss of adipose tissue. Lipodystrophies can be either congenital or acquired in origin and, depending on the extent and distribution of fat loss, are broadly categorised as generalised or partial. The severity of the metabolic complications of lipodystrophy such as T2DM, dyslipidaemia and NAFLD are roughly proportional to the extent of lipoatrophy [1]. Congenital generalised lipodystrophy is usually present at birth, and is typically associated with severe metabolic problems during childhood. Familial partial lipodystrophies (FPLD) manifest variable degrees of lipoatrophy, most frequently affecting the lower limbs and femorogluteal fat depots, and often only become clinically apparent during puberty in girls or even later in boys [1].

A combination of positional cloning and candidate gene-based sequencing approaches has resulted in the identification of ten different monogenic causes of lipodystrophies to date [1]. These lipodystrophies are currently classified on the basis of the identified genes harbouring the causative mutation. Although detailed molecular understanding of the link between the mutations and the observed phenotypes remains uncertain in several cases, lipodystrophies can be mechanistically grouped as follows: (1) genes/proteins implicated in the regulation of adipocyte differentiation – peroxisome proliferator-activated receptor-γ *(PPARG)*, lamin A/C *(LMNA)*, zinc metalloprotease *(ZMPSTE24)*, Berardinelli-Seip congenital lipodystrophy 2 *(BSCL2)* and v-AKT murine thymoma oncogene homolog 2 *(AKT2)*; (2) genes/proteins implicated in the regulation of triglyceride (TAG) synthesis – 1-acylglycerol-3-phosphate -O-acyltransferase 2 (*AGPAT2*), or (3) genes/proteins implicated in the regulation of cellular fatty acid uptake – caveolin 1 *(CAV1)* and polymerase I and transcript release factor *(PTRF)* [2]. The fact that all of the genes/proteins above are expressed in a range of cell types/tissues in addition to adipocytes has raised interesting, and for the most part unresolved, questions about the apparently tissue selective phenotypes observed and the relative contribution of mutant protein (e.g. PPARG) expression in tissues other than fat.

Lipid Droplet Proteins and Lipodystrophy

White adipose tissue (WAT) is the major energy storage organ for all vertebrates, and functions to buffer postprandial energy flux and release of non-esterified fatty acids for oxidation by other oxidative tissues in response to fasting or exercise [3]. Individual adipocytes within WAT store fat in a specialised organelle, the lipid droplet (LD), which occupies up to 90% of the cell's volume in a mature adipocyte. LDs consist of a neutral lipid core, mainly triacylglycerol and cholesterol ester, coated by a monolayer of phospholipids and associated LD proteins. Several studies suggest that as many as 200 proteins may be involved in the regulation of LD formation and breakdown [4]; however, only a small subset of these are selectively present in adipocytes where they presumably perform unique biological functions [5].

Given the central role played by adipocytes and more specifically LD proteins in regulating lipid storage and lipid flux into and out of adipocytes, we hypothesised that loss-of-function mutations in adipose-selective LD proteins might be involved in causing lipodystrophy and other related metabolic problems. In order to test this hypothesis, we proceeded to sequence the coding regions of adipocyte LD proteins/genes. This approach subsequently led to the identification of mutations in cell death-inducing DNA fragmentation factor-α-like effector c *(CIDEC)* and perilipin 1 *(PLIN1)* in patients with novel subtypes of familial partial lipodystrophy [6, 7].

Cell Death-Inducing DNA Fragmentation Factor-α-Like Effector C

CIDEC is a LD protein required for the formation of large, unilocular LDs in adipocytes. Recent cellular studies have demonstrated that Cidec overexpression increases LD size, whilst knockdown of Cidec decreased LD size and increased LD number [8, 9]. Deletion of the murine homologue of CIDEC, often referred to as Fsp27 (fat-specific protein of 27 kDa), results in reduced WAT mass, resistance to diet-induced obesity and enhanced insulin sensitivity [10, 11]. Furthermore, Fsp27-deficient mice harbour adipocytes bearing small multilocular LDs [10, 11].

Sequencing the CIDEC gene in patients with unexplained congenital lipodystrophy led to the identification of a novel homozygous non-sense mutation in CIDEC [6]. The CIDEC E186X mutation is predicted to result in premature truncation of the C-terminal portion of the protein, and cellular studies showed that the CIDEC mutant protein fails to localise to LDs and to promote an increase in LD size. Adipose tissue histology from one patient with the CIDEC E186X mutation revealed adipocytes of smaller size with increased mitochondrial content. Most strikingly, many white adipocytes in a tissue sample from the CIDEC E186X patient exhibited a remarkable multilocular LD phenotype. These data are in agreement with observations from mouse and cellular knockout models, but in contrast to the mouse Fsp27 knockout model, the patient with the CIDEC mutation manifested an adverse lipodystrophic phenotype including severe IR, T2DM, dyslipidaemia and NAFLD [6].

Perilipin 1

Perilipin 1 is the most abundant adipocyte LD coat protein, and is required for optimal TAG metabolism [12]. Two independent groups described the perilipin (Plin1)-null mouse phenotype as lean and resistant to obesity [13, 14]. In addition, perilipin-null mice exhibited increased basal lipolysis but diminished catecholamine-stimulated lipolysis. Conversely, overexpression of perilipin 1 increased TAG storage, inhibited basal lipolysis and enhanced catecholamine-stimulated lipolysis in cellular models [13–15]. These data collectively suggest that perilipin function is essential for optimal metabolic regulation of TAG metabolism in adipocytes.

We recently reported two novel heterozygous loss-of-function *PLIN1* mutations (p.398fs and p.404fs) in patients with a novel subtype of partial familial lipodystrophy, subsequently designated as familial partial lipodystrophy type 4 or FPLD4 [7]. Both mutations affect the C-terminus of the protein and coincidently result in incorporation of almost identical (one has 6 more amino acids than the other, but the rest of the amino acids are identical) aberrant amino acids from the frameshift position. Both mutations co-segregated with partial lipodystrophy, IR, hepatic steatosis and dyslipidaemia in three French families. Although the phenotypic information is currently based on a total of only 6 affected subjects, initial clinical assessment suggests that in this particular form of FPLD, the fat loss is partial throughout all adipose depots in the body.

Histological analysis of patient adipose tissue biopsies revealed a reduction in adipocyte size as well as increased macrophage infiltration and significant adipose tissue fibrosis. Cellular characterisation of mutant protein function revealed reduced ability of the mutant forms of perilipin 1 to promote TAG storage or to increase LD size when overexpressed in 3T3-L1 preadipocytes, which lack endogenous perilipin. Both mutants failed to inhibit basal lipolysis when overexpressed 3T3-L1 preadipocytes. In addition, patients and stably transfected cells manifest lower levels of mutant protein expression, which could also contribute to the observed cellular phenotype. Further investigation suggested a specific cellular mechanism for the increase in basal lipolysis [16]. Adipose TAG lipase (ATGL) is the major lipase responsible for the initial step in TAG hydrolysis in adipocytes, and is required for basal lipolysis [17]. Perilipin 1 reduces basal lipolysis by indirectly regulating ATGL activity. It does this by binding and sequestering α/β hydrolase domain-containing protein 5 (ABHD5), an ATGL coactivator [18]. By employing bimolecular fluorescence complementation assays, we demonstrated that both perilipin frameshift mutants fail to bind ABHD5 and prevent its interaction with ATGL, thus increasing ATGL activity and basal lipolysis [16].

Conclusions

Although it is widely accepted that obesity is the most prevalent cause of human IR and ultimately T2DM, several studies in patients with insulin-resistant T2DM have suggested that defects in insulin-stimulated glucose uptake in muscle and the ability to suppress hepatic glucose output are the predominant mechanisms underpinning the development of IR [19]. In some non-obese patients, these would appear to be primary events in the pathogenesis of T2DM, and it has even been suggested that they could cause weight gain. Lipodystrophic patients, particularly those with mutations in CIDEC and PLIN1, which are almost exclusively expressed in adipocytes, provide compelling evidence for the primary role of adipose tissue dysfunction in at least some forms of IR.

Free fatty acids released from adipocytes as a consequence of increased basal lipolysis are thought to precipitate macrophage recruitment and accumulation within adipose tissue. An elegant rodent study by Kosteli et al. [20] recently provided compelling evidence for the primary role of locally released free fatty acids in prompting macrophage recruitment into adipose tissue. Perturbations which promoted adipocyte lipolysis increased macrophage numbers in WAT, whereas ATGL knockdown prevented this response and alleviated IR [20]. The similarities we observed in terms of macrophage accumulation and fibrosis in WAT from patients with the PLIN1 mutations are consistent with these findings [7]. Intriguingly, both perilipin and CIDEC mRNA expression levels were found to be lower in WAT samples from obese insulin-resistant people than in samples from obese insulin-sensitive controls [21], implying that what we observed in patients with loss-of-function mutations in these two LD proteins may also pertain to more prevalent forms of IR.

Lipodystrophy is a rare cause of extreme IR and T2DM, but progress in understanding the molecular basis of this cluster of disorders has informed our understanding of adipocyte biology and, perhaps more importantly, highlighted the devastating systemic consequences of a mismatch between energy intake and the capacity to safely store surplus energy as triacylglycerol in adipocyte LDs. This mismatch is clearly extreme in lipodystrophy, but is also thought to be a core feature of obesity-associated IR where sustained positive energy balance ultimately appears to result in lipid overflow to ectopic sites such as the liver and skeletal muscle where it is widely implicated in causing IR and T2DM [19].

Acknowledgements

Our work in this area is supported by grants from the Wellcome Trust, the UK NIHR Cambridge Biomedical Research Centre, the UK Medical Research Council Centre for Obesity and Related Metabolic Diseases and the Clinical Research Infrastructure Grant.

References

1 Garg A: Lipodystrophies: Genetic and acquired body fat disorders. J Clin Endocrinol Metab 2011; 96:3313–3325.

2 Garg A, Agarwal AK: Lipodystrophies: Disorders of adipose tissue biology. Biochim Biophys Acta 2009; 1791:507–513.

3 Frayn KF: Adipose tissue as a buffer for daily lipid flux. Diabetologia 2002;45:1201–1210.

4 Guo Y, Walther TC, Rao M, Stuurman N, Goshima G, Terayama K, et al: Functional genomic screen reveals genes involved in lipid-droplet formation and utilization. Nature 2008;453:657–661.

5 Farese RV Jr, Walther TC: Lipid droplets finally get a little R-E-S-P-E-C-T. Cell 2009;139:855–860.

6 Rubio-Cabezas O, Puri V, Murano I, Saudek V, Semple RK, Dash S, et al: Partial lipodystrophy and insulin resistant diabetes in a patient with a homozygous nonsense mutation in CIDEC. EMBO Mol Med 2009;1:280–287.

7 Gandotra S, Le Dour C, Bottomley W, Cervera P, Giral P, Reznik Y, et al: Perilipin deficiency and autosomal dominant partial lipodystrophy. N Engl J Med 2011;364:740–748.

8 Keller P, Petrie JT, De Rose P, Gerin I, Wright WS, Chiang S-H, et al: Fat-specific protein 27 regulates storage of triacylglycerol. J Biol Chem 2008;283: 14355–14365.

9 Puri V, Konda S, Ranjit S, Aouadi M, Chawla A, Chouinard M, et al: Fat-specific protein 27, a novel lipid droplet protein that enhances triglyceride storage. J Biol Chem 2007;282:34213–34218.

10 Nishino N, Tamori Y, Tateya S, Kawaguchi T, Shibakusa T, Mizunoya W, et al: FSP27 contributes to efficient energy storage in murine white adipocytes by promoting the formation of unilocular lipid droplets. J Clin Invest 2008;118:2808–2821.

11 Toh SY, Gong J, Du G, Li JZ, Yang S, Ye J, et al: Upregulation of mitochondrial activity and acquirement of brown adipose tissue-like property in the white adipose tissue of Fsp27 deficient mice. PLoS ONE 2008;3:e2890.

12 Bickel PE, Tansey JT, Welte MA: PAT proteins, an ancient family of lipid droplet proteins that regulate cellular lipid stores. Biochim Biophys Acta 2009; 1791:419–440.

13 Martinez-Botas J, Anderson JB, Tessier D, Lapillonne A, Chang BH-J, Quast MJ, et al: Absence of perilipin results in leanness and reverses obesity in Leprdb/db mice. Nat Genet 2000;26:474–479.

14 Tansey JT, Sztalryd C, Gruia-Gray J, Roush DL, Zee JV, Gavrilova O, et al: Perilipin ablation results in a lean mouse with aberrant adipocyte lipolysis, enhanced leptin production, and resistance to diet-induced obesity. Proc Natl Acad Scie 2001;98: 6494–6499.

15 Brasaemle D, Subramanian V, Garcia A, Marcinkiewicz A, Rothenberg A: Perilipin A and the control of triacylglycerol metabolism. Mol Cell Biochem 2009;326:15–21.

16 Gandotra S, Lim K, Girousse A, Saudek V, O'Rahilly S, Savage DB: Human frameshift mutations affecting the carboxyl terminus of perilipin increase lipolysis by failing to sequester the adipose triglyceride lipase (ATGL) coactivator, AB-hydrolase containing 5 (ABHD5). J Biol Chem 2011;286: 34998–35006.

17 Zimmermann R, Strauss JG, Haemmerle G, Schoiswohl G, Birner-Gruenberger R, Riederer M, et al: Fat mobilization in adipose tissue is promoted by adipose triglyceride lipase. Science 2004;306:1383–1386.

18 Granneman JG, Moore H-PH, Krishnamoorthy R, Rathod M: Perilipin controls lipolysis by regulating the interactions of AB-hydrolase containing 5 (Abhd5) and adipose triglyceride lipase (Atgl). J Biol Chem 2009;284:34538–34544.

19 Savage DB, Petersen KF, Shulman GI: Disordered lipid metabolism and the pathogenesis of insulin resistance. Physiol Rev 2007;87:507–520.

20 Kosteli A, Sugaru E, Haemmerle G, Martin JF, Lei J, Zechner R, et al: Weight loss and lipolysis promote a dynamic immune response in murine adipose tissue. J Clin Invest 2010;120:3466–3479.

21 Puri V, Ranjit S, Konda S, Nicoloro SMC, Straubhaar J, Chawla A, et al: Cidea is associated with lipid droplets and insulin sensitivity in humans. Proc Natl Acad Sci 2008;105:7833–7838.

Dr. David B. Savage
Metabolic Research Laboratories, Institute of Metabolic Science
University of Cambridge, Addenbrooke's Hospital
Hills Road, Cambridge CB2 0QQ (UK)
E-Mail dbs23@medschl.cam.ac.uk

Author Index

Subject Index